The Power Lies In You

An Epic Guide to Regenerative Self-Care

Brooke Nicole, MPH

The Power Lies In You
Copyright © 2021 Brooke Nicole, MPH

The resources in this book are provided for informational purposes only and should not be used to replace the specialized training and professional judgment of your health care or mental health care professional.

The author disclaims responsibility for adverse effects or consequences from the misapplication or injudicious use of the information contained in this book.

Cover Design by Jennifer Rae

ISBN: 979-8-9854251-0-9

CONTENTS

Foreword

My first time meeting Brooke, I was taken with her pure passion, her quiet thoughtfulness and her determination. I was impressed with her commitment and intentionality around homeschooling her children and inspired by the way she lives her life, full of experience, community, contribution and faith.

She stopped by a few months later, her children in tow, to deliver the most thoughtful gift basket. It was full of local products she purchased with her family and was thoughtfully arranged. But her presence and the incredible behavior of her young children were what left the biggest impression on me.

When she left, I sat and reflected on the beautiful force of this quiet woman I had just spent time with. How do I make changes in my life to be more grounded and at peace like she exuded? How do I help my children feel so confidant, calm and also beautifully behaved? And how can I be a thoughtful gift giver like she is?

Fortunately, The Power Lies In You is a guide to do exactly that. To become the most connected version of you through care of self. To simplify your life in a way that is intentional and rewarding. To focus on what is important and to navigate what it means to be healthy, physically and mentally, without the overwhelm.

The gem of a book you are about to read is truly about care of self, something that is missing from so many of our lives. We are constantly looking outside of ourselves, hoping to buy the peace we so desperately crave. Settle in, you're about to unlearn what true self-care is.

Growing up on a farm, in a community of hardworking rural Americans, luxuries like spas, expensive products or gym memberships seemed wasteful and indulgent. I prided myself on low maintenance living. Until I got a taste of my first professional massage that worked the knots out of a summer of double shifts waitressing to earn tuition money for college.

I was hooked. And as I applied the work ethic that I'd seen modeled by my parents to my corporate job, I earned the income that allowed for those luxuries I'd grown up judging. As self-care became en vogue, mani pedis and massages were scheduled in and honored, even when my daily workouts weren't.

One day, I had a realization. I was rushing straight from work (leaving at 7pm) to a massage appointment I was usually late for, not even giving myself time to relax in the steam shower prior. I was paying for an hour of quiet, of disconnecting to reconnect to myself. For the first 30 min, I'd have racing thoughts before finally falling asleep, only to wake up slightly irritated that I hadn't really "experienced" the relaxation.

It was more than a decade later that I realized that the peace, the self-care and the connection I was seeking wasn't found in a monthly massage or quarterly spa day. Though I still love a bit of pampering, the truth lies in the elements of how we construct our daily life, in the practices that weave the fabric of our experience.

In truly understanding your needs to be the most whole and happy version of yourself, you can identify your non-negotiables for being you. At the beginning of 2020, when the world was upended and stress and anxiety were so easy to find, I wrote this list out of my basic needs for maintaining my sanity and happiness.

When I separated my needs versus wants, I was taken with how short the list was, and how simple it really was to fulfill each day.

Healthy, nourishing foods

Connection time with loved ones

Time in nature

Movement

I realized that I could take my children outside for a hike in nature or to the beach and we could combine movement, time in nature and connection. At the end of the hour or so outside, we were happy, tired out and connected. It was simple, and required no screens, toys or money.

A year later, I realized there was one more missing element that you will discover in The Power Lies in You. It's simple, but please, don't minimize its power. Time to yourself and the focus on breath.

Over the years, I've dabbled with different morning routines, trying to find the perfect combination that would result in me feeling inspired for my day, focused and energetic. No combo quite delivered in under an hour (a necessity with small children who seemed uniquely able to sense when I was deep in meditation and wake up then!).

I was introduced to a tool of breath work, one that combines breath work, meditation and visioning that I craved making my morning non-negotiable. Reconnecting me back to myself, daily breath work has made me more connected, trust myself and my intuition more, be in more aligned action, waste less time, be more patient and connected with my family and have confidence in my ability to commit to something and honor it. When I'm disconnected from going within, is when I go outwards for validation or fulfillment. And it never works.

Wherever you are when you read this, give yourself permission to do less to be more. Commit, or recommit, to a few simple practices that will give you more peace, good health and happiness.

After reading and digesting The Power Lies In You, I commit to:

- Shopping from local farmers markets - I spent six weeks in Europe and fell in love with buying groceries every other day, seeing what I found in season, being beckoned by the most beautiful or fragrant offerings. Food had never tasted fresher, even when the meals were so simple. I recommit to supporting the local economy and reducing my carbon footprint by shopping in season at the nearby farmers market.

- Growing my own herbs to share with my children to share my experience growing up eating from my own garden. Seeing them go out and eat fresh mint while playing outside makes me SO happy.

- Taking my children into nature, daily. I've often pondered, how do I give my children more of the outdoor education and nature appreciation I grew up with, that I've disconnected from? Camping, hiking, beach time with toes in the sand.... so they can have an appreciation and love for the earth we live on. In nature, the world becomes an experience and your imagination is all you require... no need for toys or figuring out activities to amuse your children.

- Focusing on intentional giving. This year, instead of making an income goal for my business, I made a giving goal, not just monetarily, but also in the energy and time I wanted to give back each month.

I so look forward to see what you commit to, how you become more connected to yourself and how you practice your sustainable care of self. When we are conscious of ourselves and what we nourish ourselves with, we become more conscious of our connection with the whole, to other humans, to the beauty of the earth and its gifts.

This book is one of those gifts.

CHAPTER I

It's Time To Change

"Change is the fear of the unknown.
But if you don't change, you don't grow."

– DR. EDITH EVA EGER

Maybe you've done this too. Your free-spirited little child self believed that you could fly. So you climb onto the tallest branch that you can in your most favorite tree with your heart pounding so loud in your chest while you stretch out your arms wide, close your eyes, and then jump. You imagine that you are soaring to the utmost heights until you realize that the force of gravity is stronger than your most powerful imaginations and you brace yourself for the unhappy landing.

I was completely devastated by the fact that I could not fly. Yet, because of this devastation, I became aware of the fact that I do *NOT* possess superpower abilities like a superhero cartoon character.

It became apparent that the power lies in me to realize that although I may not possess superpower abilities, my unique gifts and talents can be used to do powerful things if I focus on what I can do instead of what I cannot do. I still to this day cannot fly, but what I am certain that I can do today is *BE* the best person I can by using the capabilities and talents that I am blessed with.

That day I chose to use the power that lies in me to use the gifts and talents that I am graced with to the utmost of my ability.

This is called conviction. You first have to be convicted with the fact that even though you may not have the power to fly from a tree, the power lies in you to see your true potential and use your unique capabilities in ways that you only can.

It is no mistake that you are here. You have been put here on this earth because you have an unequivocal purpose to make this world a beautiful place, whether or not you can fly. You are precious beyond measure, valued, and honored. You have a passion to make this world a better place, and the power lies in you to realize that.

Do you believe that?

A blind boy sat on the steps of a building with a hat by his feet. He held up a sign which read, "I am blind, please help." There were only a few coins in the hat with spare change from folks as they hurried past.

A man was walking by. He took a few coins from his pocket and dropped them into the hat. He then took the sign, turned it around, and wrote some words. Then he put the sign back into the boy's hand so that everyone who walked by would see the new words.

Soon the hat began to fill up. A lot more people were giving money to the blind boy. That afternoon, the man who had changed the sign returned to see how things were. The boy recognized his footsteps and asked, "Were you the one who changed my sign this morning? What did you write?" The man said, "I only wrote the truth. I said what you said but differently." I wrote, "Today is a beautiful day, but I cannot see it."

Both signs spoke the truth. But the first sign simply said that the boy was blind, while the second sign conveyed to everyone walking by how grateful they should be to see.

No matter what you are experiencing at this present moment, whether it may seem as though you have darkness surrounding you or familiarity with the many pleasures of this life, the power lies in you to *change* the sign that you have written on yourself. And in doing so, you will change your life and the lives of others.

Just like this blind boy, the problem is that most people label themselves below what their true capability is and do not see the reality that the power is actually in them to make a change in their small realm of influence. The blind boy held the changed sign that helped others see the blessings that they had, while in return receiving the blessing that he was looking for all along, more than what he expected.

That blind boy experienced regenerative self-care. His sign needed to first be changed from the common fact to the unexpected truth to receive what he was looking for. In appreciation for the truthful sign in the blind boy's hand, the people walking by began to be grateful for the reality that they could see the beautiful day, and their gratitude, in return, benefited that blind boys need.

Self-care must help you to become the person you want to be and fulfill your needs beyond what you even anticipated. If you are not experiencing this, then you are doing self-care all wrong.

Regenerative self-care gives back, is perpetual, and restores you and others as a whole.

Time after time I would get a spa treatment in hopes that the enormous amount of money that I spent would give me the relaxation I needed for at least one week, but by the next day, I needed another one. It is because of this reality that there is a myth that to enjoy self-care, you have to be wealthy.

Self-care isn't something that you do 30 minutes a day, twice a month, or once a year. Regenerative self-care is a lifestyle that is made up of powerful moment-by-moment choices. And those choices become a part of who you are.

I am here to tell you that you do not have to own a country in your bank account to experience sustaining relief that self-care provides. Right now, you can live regenerative self-care by changing the way that you view yourself from your past label. This is the first step.

It's time to change the sign that you have been holding. It's time to understand the need to take care of yourself in a way that can bless others in the process of fulfilling your need. It all starts with your view.

WHAT YOU THOUGHT THEN

Being the youngest of three girls in my family, I had a lot to live up to. One had the brain, the other had the beauty, and I possessed the title of getting away with things. Some would call that spoiled. I do have to admit that I did take advantage of that title to the nth degree, yet my sign that I held of myself was just stating that I could get away with things.

Sure, I was able to do things that my sisters may not have been able to do, but that did not bring sustaining happiness. Because of the way that I viewed myself from the title that I learned in my early years, I could not see any potential beyond that title. It was the stagnant truth and that became who I was.

I had a label and I began to believe that there was nothing I could do to change that fact. I began defining myself as one who could get away with a lot of things, not have to work hard to get things, and therefore not receive the joy from the choices I made or any hard work that I put forth. My life and outlook felt like that blind boy with his first sign and just enough coins in his hat to get by.

What you think affects the way that you feel. The way you feel is shown by your behaviors and actions. Your actions lead to your character, and how you view your character leads to the belief in your true potential.

The power lies in you to change the way that you think of yourself and transform those labels that may hinder you from becoming the real you.

You have the powerful choice to live the life that you are intended to live. There is only one catch. Change has to happen. Change the way that you were, and reimagine the person you want to become.

I was once asked, "What do you want to be when you grow up?" A typical answer was spewed out of my mouth. I wanted to be a firefighter. Today, I am not a firefighter because I asked myself 'why'. My answer to why I did not want to become a firefighter did not completely resonate with who I wanted to become. Your views, goals, and convictions may change, but the power that lies in you to obtain your true honor and usefulness in your unique capability does not change.

Your views that you had of yourself when you were young may have had a huge role in playing out how you are today. Do not take that for granted. Yet, take this time to truly ask yourself how accurate those views are with who you are today.

• **What was the view that you had of yourself when you were young?**

_____

_____

_____

_____

ASK YOURSELF

14

• **Did you ever feel like the view of yourself did not resonate with who you really were?**

_____

_____

_____

_____

• **How did it affect the way that you grew up?**

_____

_____

_____

_____

HOW TO CHANGE YOUR SIGN

I don't know about you, but I for sure wanted to change my childhood sign to correctly portray my message to align with the person who I had changed into as an adult. There is always room for improvement and there is definite fear in change. What will people think? What if people do not see the change? What if I am not good enough? Change is done by actions. So to alleviate your fear, make small additions to achieve your desired result.

One small step that I added to my life once I realized that I wanted to change my sign, was adopting the acronym V.I.P.

V- View.

Your view is your outlook on life, your convictions, and how you perceive yourself. Does your current view of yourself help you accomplish who you want to be in the long run? What story do you want to write for your life? Who do you desire to be that you aren't living at this moment in time? It may be difficult to think of a long-term dream, so begin by looking two years down the road. What do you want to accomplish in that period of time? As you think of your story and how you want it to be written, be S.M.A.R.T. when thinking of your view and vision, for this will help you identify explicitly what you want to achieve.

S.pecific

M.easurable

A.ctionable

R.ealistic

T.imebound

I- Inspiration.

How do you inspire yourself to see how much you have changed from the past and continue to strive to be even better? Is it through writing post-it notes on your bathroom mirror, breaking your goal into smaller parts, or doing something that makes you happy first like listening to music, reading, or exercising?

P- Positive Pattern.

Who is someone that exemplifies a pattern that you want to model? Look at their character qualities, lifestyle habits, and outlook on life and apply those patterns to your own.

Think about where you are now and what sign you are holding. Ask yourself, "Is my sign correctly portraying to others my message that I desire to get across that is in alignment with who I am at this present moment? Am I purposefully seeking to benefit and bless myself and others?"

Who do you want to become? Do you want to experience more joy? Live a more fulfilled life? Experience more successes? How does the way that you viewed yourself when you were young affect you from becoming who you want to be now? The power lies in you to change your life and others around you. You just have to be willing to make the change from what was, to what is.

As you think about this, take a moment to write your vision for yourself if it is any different than when you were young.

• **What is the story that you want for yourself?**

_____

_____

_____

_____

WRITE IT

• **What view or vision do you have for yourself in the next two years? Incorporate S.M.A.R.T. into that view.**

_____

_____

_____

_____

• **How will you inspire yourself to change your label?**

_____

_____

_____

- **Who is someone that exemplifies a pattern that you want to model and why?**

_____

_____

_____

WHAT YOU THINK NOW

During my Master of Public Health coursework, I became acquainted with cognitive distorted thinking and my mind was blown away with this one simple concept. How can something so simple like changing the way you think solve major problems with how you view yourself?

This was something that I immediately began applying to the way that I was labeled as the one who got away with things. Over time, my distorted thinking from how I was labeled began to be reframed to believe that although I may have been placed with that label, the power lies in me to change my view in accordance with who I am. The power lies in me to believe that I am capable of being valued. The power lies in me to choose to use this experience to encourage others.

When my view became correct alongside my current temperament, values, and outlook on life, it was as though I had permitted myself to live the life that I was intended to live. There was no pressure to live in a box that was stamped by others' opinions and views. And might I add, this permission to live the life that you are intended to live is not to label yourself below what you are capable of, yet to give you the ability and opportunity to fully shine the gifts and talents that only you are graced with.

• **What is the view that you have of yourself now?**

_____

_____

_____

_____

ASK YOURSELF

• **How is this view different than the view when you were younger?**

_____

_____

_____

_____

- **How will this view affect the way that you live your life from now on?**

_____

_____

_____

_____

WHAT IS STOPPING YOU?

It can be tough changing your view, especially if your environment hasn't changed. Even if your surroundings have not changed, you have. You're not the same person that you used to be, but only you can choose to take that first step to change the sign that has been hindering you from living that reality.

Do you now believe me when I tell you that you are precious, valued, and honored? That only you have a special message that the world needs to hear? That the power lies in _YOU_ to improve your well-being by creating an honest and healthy outlook, reducing harmful imbalances, and incorporating sufficient time to recharge?

Learn how to embrace the value of who you are and live a life that is restored, recharged, renewed, and purposeful instead of one that is life-sucking and temporarily filled.

Knowing, breathing, and living your changed view of yourself gives you renewed energy. This change can intrigue you with power and inspire you to do something about it.

As your view has changed, so will the way that you take care of yourself. The term self-care will bring about a whole new way of thinking as you live your day-to-day life. You will begin to encounter regenerative self-care holistically and you can set about to enjoy your hat full of coins in return.

To make change, you must first find value in the change. Recognize something has to be done to make the change. Make the effort to change. And do all in your power to keep the change moving.

The power lies in you to start living regenerative self-care today by:

Changing your past labels.

Reliving your past experiences and filing them away.

Learning how to make focused action that aligns with who you are.

Restoring your mind-body connection.

Eating for the benefit of others.

Shifting the way you live to help the environment.

Choosing your company to help you become the person you want to be.

If you want to change the way that you self-care, let me begin to share with you how regenerative self-care not just begins with your changed view, but how the power lies in you to change the way self-care is done.

Let's give self-care a new look.

CHAPTER 2

Rewrite Your Story

"One's life story cannot be told with complete veracity. A true autobiography would have to be written in states of mind, emotions, heartbeats, smiles and tears; not in months and years, or physical events. Life is marked off on the soul by feelings, not by dates."

– HELEN KELLER

For self-care to be given a new look, your story has to be rewritten. We are all human, and we all have a story that has made us the way that we are today. The powerful thing about your life story is that instead of being the author of your unhappiness, you get to rewrite your story while you are still alive that will open up opportunities to change the final ending.

My story began to be rewritten when one day I had a wake-up call. Looking back, it was pretty funny how it all happened, yet I am forever thankful for it.

When I was pregnant with my firstborn, I found myself on the ground, not because I was in a transcendent state, but because I didn't know how I got there. All I wanted was a drink of water, but the doorframe had proven victor as I lay there wondering what had just happened.

After a few moments, I became fully aware that my thoughts were on a long time wound that was never healed. Something had triggered my subconscious mind and as I lay there on the ground, my life tape rewound to when I was a little girl.

It was a warm day, yet I remember the vivid feeling of becoming cold and sensing aloofness as I walked through the house. I was looking for my Dad and he was nowhere to be found. I thought, "He's not anywhere in the house, let me check in the garage since I haven't looked there yet." I opened the garage door and there he was, I had found him. Just not how I was expecting.

There was a rope that hung from the roof of the garage and it was wrapped around my Dad's neck.

In a shaky voice I asked him, "What are you doing, Daddy?" He only replied with a blank stare. Not knowing what to do, after a few seemingly long moments, I closed the door and retreated to my room in what felt like ten million steps walking through quicksand.

What I thought then in my little girl's mind was, "You don't need me? Then I don't need you." I still remember the feeling of my heart hardening as I did my best to process what I had just experienced. This began the unknowingly long journey to find self-care that would heal my heart and mind.

The self-care habits that I began to partake in from that day on were binge eating, relationships, and searching in all the wrong places for that stripped away peace. When all of these short-term 'joys' had ended, I was in no different place than when I started.

My Dad did not take his life that day, and each day seeing him seemed to make it harder to cope and find the alignment that I once had.

As the days went on, this incident was never talked about. When I was in college, I concluded that he should know what he did to me. So, I took the opportunity to yell at him, cry angry tears at him, demand him to say sorry for what he had done, and blame him for the unhappiness that I had experienced for all of my life. I thought that by doing this, I would feel better and my happiness and love for him would return.

It did not happen as I had hoped, but the pivotal point in my journey was my Dad's reaction to my crazy irrationalness. He listened quietly for over an hour, then when I demanded him to say something, all he said was, "I love you, I am sorry."

Even though I knew that he was sincere and poured every ounce of love into those words, I did not forgive my Dad that day.

My Dad's death came quickly, and now that he was gone, the guilt overwhelmed me that I did not say, "I forgive you" while he was still alive. I was crushed by the fact that I stole joy from him all those years due to my pride believing that it was his fault for my unhappiness, not mine. All of this now rested upon my heavy heart as I was at his bedside as he passed.

After my Dad's death, instead of using the power of my vulnerability at that moment to forgive, I used it to harbor more anger towards him and more sympathy to myself instead. The worst part of it all, I acted like everything was fine while I went on with my life. That's how I coped from the very beginning, so it only made sense to do it once again.

Now, here I was on the ground five years after my Dad passed away because I still had not forgiven him. I had not dealt with the problem and it was stealing my happiness, and therefore not allowing me to live to the true potential that I was capable of at that moment. Because of that doorframe, I was then determined to bury the hatchet and end this pain once and for all. For sure, I did not want to steal any happiness from my soon-to-be-born child because of my past negative experiences.

I got up from the floor, rubbed my belly, and went to the kitchen to get the drink of water that I was intending to get in the first place. That drink of water was the sweetest that I have ever tasted.

It was not until seven years after my Dad passed away that I was truly free from the pride and guilt that my non-forgiving attitude had produced all those years.

It took two years for me to process and change my thoughts to a forgiving one after that doorframe knocked me down, but it doesn't have to take that long. That doorframe knocked some sense into me and put me on a forgiveness journey that began to change my life, slowly might I add, because I had a lot of pride to knock off.

The first question I began to ask myself was, "why didn't I have forgiveness for my Dad when he told me that he was sorry?" This could have been dealt with so much earlier and had prevented so much heartache and unnecessary pain.

That forthright wake-up call helped me to rewrite my life story so that I could heal on an emotional level and thrive on a mental level. Forgiving your past has a powerful way of bringing clarity in your life and rebuilding your foundation of trust that you may have lost. No one but yourself can compel you to forgive, yet it is this power that lies in you that can rewrite your story. The first step is the hardest.

1. **Chuck your pride out the window.**
    The first and hardest realization is admitting that you need to forgive.

Pride must be put away. Even though someone may say they are sorry by their words or actions, there is a tendency for pride to not allow you to forgive because you may justify that it is easy to say 'I'm sorry', but it does not make everything right.

Forgiving someone does not mean forgetting what was done, but it allows you to let go of your pride in holding on to the past event, that you cannot change.

2. **Put the other persons' shoes on.**
    In order to understand the other person, we must put their shoes on and see things from their perspective.

Before I was born, my dad had an industrial accident that was life-threatening with a prognosis of only living a few months. He miraculously survived and lived over 30 years after that doctor's prediction, but from that, he become a type one diabetic from damage to his pancreas and other internal organs. His medications later caused him to become deaf and after several years he was chronically in pain.

He was constantly in the hospital for either his blood sugar episodes or him receiving pain medication. Living that type of life can be one that wears a person down. Growing up, I always thought that I was the one who had to suffer because most times we were woken up in the middle of the night because we were too young to stay home alone, and we ended up sleeping in the hospital waiting room chairs. I could have kept a pillow there for our frequent visits. But when I saw things from his perspective, my walls of pride began to crumble and I began to feel sympathetic towards him in what he really had to go through.

When I would ask him how his pain felt, he would say it's like being punched in the solar plexus x10. I have been punched in the solar plexus, and it sure did not feel good. Not for a while, either, which then made me understand just a portion of the pain that he had to experience day in and day out.

Even though thinking to take one's life is not a healthy solution to any problem, I could see how my dad was looking for some type of relief from his constant pain.

Seeing things from another person's perspective does not excuse any wrong or harmful act, but it can allow you to make more sense of why an action may have been done.

3. Determine that you want a life of happiness.
A life of happiness is the belief that this moment is all that you have and live to its fullest.

Trying to change the past or worrying about the future only distracts you from what is truly important... living now! To not be present in the moment is to lose that moment in time forever.

This is not to be confused with remembering how the past has led you to where you are today and learning from those mistakes, nor from looking ahead to the future and having a plan in place for how you will overcome your obstacles.

When my dad's death came suddenly, I had an overwhelming sense of guilt that I had stolen happiness from him and myself that we both could have enjoyed. And now, that opportunity was gone forever.

Choose today that you will embrace every moment. For the days may be long, but the years quick. Stop to notice how your daughter twirls her hair around her finger, listen to the expressed joys of your son, draw close to your partner and feel their heartbeat, call your mother, give food to someone who is hungry. Do things today that you will not regret tomorrow, for tomorrow is not guaranteed.

4. Train your mind.
You have to change your thoughts or actions of hurt to a

31

loving and accepting attitude.

Even though this is the final step, this is the second hardest step in your forgiveness journey, apart from the first step in putting your pride away. It is realizing that you still have negative feelings towards your event and/or individual when it may come up again and again.

I could not understand why I kept feeling hurt and angry when stories of my dad were told or why I didn't want to visit his graveside. Hadn't I already forgiven him? Why was I still feeling negative towards the situation?

I began to realize that forgiveness is not just saying 'I forgive you', neither is being sorry just saying, 'I'm sorry'. It is an entire action that you have to train your mind to make new positive pathways that redirect your negative thoughts and actions. When you say I'm sorry, you have to change your action from what you are sorry from to something acceptable so that you truly mean that you will not do it again.

It is the same thing with forgiveness. You have to change your thoughts or actions of hurt to a loving and accepting attitude, but that does not come overnight.

Your brain activates a certain feeling from what it has been trained to do each time that event comes up. And for all those years I trained my mind to think negatively towards my Dad for stealing my joy and happiness by thinking that I was not important enough for him to live for. So, even though I had gone through all of my previous steps successfully, I had to rewire the pathways of my mind from those negative feelings to positive ones.

To do that, whenever anger would come back or a negative feeling would arise, I would continuously implement the first three steps then replace that thought with a positive memory that I had of my Dad. Over time, the positive memories crowded out the negative ones and a new positive pathway of feelings had emerged.

REWRITE YOUR STORY

I am telling you my forgiveness story because it is one of the hardest things to do, yet one of the most fulfilling. It was not until I had dealt with my past, that I could appropriately see my true potential.

It's like when you taste food. To get the full flavor of each item, you need to cleanse your palate by drinking water to reset your taste buds. Forgiveness is the cleanser that resets your view and life. The power lies in you to tap into that renewal so that your life can be whole once more.

You may have a forgiveness story too. It may be similar to mine, or something totally different. Whatever experiences you may have had in the past, you need to ask yourself one thing, "What is my unforgiving action stealing from me?"

Before you can even think about forgiving and go on your forgiveness journey, you need to start with the first tool. The tool of writing out the story that might not be serving you well right now. Write every detail out including how it made you feel, what it makes you feel now, what it caused you to do then, and how has it shaped you to be who you are now. Self-observation and reflection have been used as one of the main tools to facilitate natural healing after a loss.[1]

Take a few moments, or days, to write down any loss or experience that caused you to lose something in your life. Any kind. Try to remember every detail as you put your experience into writing. As you are writing, different emotions may spring up. You may need to implement the steps for forgiveness or make sure that your self-talk is seen in its true light.

After you get it all out of your system, go back and read it through again with different lenses. This time as you read and come across a negative emotion or feeling, state the fact then correct it with a new positive thought.

An example is when I was writing my story and the feeling of guilt came up as I was remembering how I did not forgive my Dad when he was alive, I immediately wrote down my corrected view as: Although I lost many precious years with my Dad due to my un-forgiveness, that experience has taught me to not hold onto a grudge no matter how big or small and to live every moment as if this were my last.

The purpose for writing all the details down is so that you can process your emotions and allow for healthy thought changes to occur. Once this is written, read, re-read, and thought changes have taken place, you can now file it away so that your anxiety can lessen knowing where you can find it in case you want to take a moment to remember what was lost, instead of continuing to relive every moment for fear of forgetting.

Write out any past life experiences that you have not forgiven with every detail that you can remember. Do this for any part of your story that you want to be rewritten: loss of joy, loss of a loved one, loss of a job, loss of financial stability, loss of respect, loss of dignity (abuse), loss of a dream, loss of a material good, or loss of health.

Try It!

ONE SIZE DOES NOT FIT ALL

We all have our own stories of how we were raised; with the joys, the pain, and the frustration. My life was forever changed when I saw my Dad in the garage with a rope tied around his neck as he contemplated taking his life.

My views about myself changed that day, and those views were not changed again until that door frame knocked me down and I began to realize that how my upbringing and how my family self-cared during those times affected my ability to self-care as I was growing up.

This event was not talked about, brought up, or emotionally

processed. Because of that, I thought that the way to take care of this experience and myself was not to talk about things, to go on with life, and just deal with it. Even though I had no other way to show me otherwise, I knew that this was not reaching my need to heal and thrive.

I was longing for connection, and it wasn't until I opened up and saw my story from a different perspective that I was able to rewrite my story. Yet, it took me many years to understand that one person's way of self-care is not mine, neither is self-care just for the weekend or an occasional treat. Because connection is what I lost when I witnessed my Dad attempt to take his life, it was connection that I was longing for all those years.

Each one of us has a completely different makeup, meaning that your unique temperament plays an important role in regenerative self-care. Ironically, your personal, emotional, and mental self-care is the beginning of it all. It's your unique experiences that shape who you are while also being the drive for what you need.

Your frame of mind can be influenced by your family culture, what your peers thought of you growing up, and how social media convinces you that you are something that you are not. With all of these influences, it is easy to get tossed around with the idea that you need to do this or that way is the right way. You can do this and that as long as you wish, but none of that matters if it does not resonate with your distinctive and unique temperament, feelings, and needs.

For some, going to the spa reaches every desire in their living being, yet the spa treatments that I would treat myself to did not last more than one day because that form of self-care did not fulfill my need. With my natural temperament being expressive, responsive, and light-hearted, I had to do trial and error to find out what self-care habits triggered my satisfaction, relief, and overall physical and mental health.

Since connection is what I had lost, it is through connection that I feel the most restored. I get the greatest pleasure and the most fulfillment when I am with my family and we are doing things together.

The first step to truly finding a regenerative self-care lifestyle is to examine what you may have lost. Then notice when you do things of the opposite nature, how does it make you feel? Does that satisfy you and bring joy to your life?

Everyone is unique and different in his or her ways and how you match your temperament with your self-care routine will transform the way that you live. Do you eat a whole box of chocolates as your way to unwind? Do you work when you're stressed or chill out in a bubble bath? Are you the life of the party or does the thought of crowds of people intimidate you? Do you accept the truth or argue the facts? Do you oftentimes think of others before yourself or do you eat the last piece of pie?

How you answer these types of questions will help you to find what is the best form of self-care for you.

If you would like to know more about your present temperament and how to choose self-care that is in sync with your personal needs, it would be my honor to guide you to find self-care habits that are in alignment with your feelings and personal needs.

CHAPTER 3

The Regenerative Process

"Success is the product of daily habits, not
once-in-a-lifetime transformations."

– JAMES CLEAR

Self-care is not necessarily one large action or behavior. It is commonly a series of small, incremental actions and behaviors that accumulate to result in better health and wellness.

Regenerative self-care is this same kind of self-care while also being the kind that benefits every other system on our planet so that all may thrive.

Now that your story is rewritten, the next chapter is easier to write. There is a renewed sense of stamina and a new understanding that it is the little things in life that make up the big successes.

For anyone who has ever had the privilege of gardening, you will notice that gardening is a lot like us. The first thing you want to do is remove any excess rocks and other unwanted debris from the soil.

This first step you have just done by changing your view on

yourself and throwing out the unwanted rocks in your life by rewriting your story.

Now that the rocks and other materials are discarded and won't get in the way of your garden, now is the time where you build a healthy foundation. To make a garden strong, it needs to be filled with good soil. Soil that is full of tiny living things called organisms.

All of these tiny living organisms that make up a healthy foundation work together for one common goal. To yield good tasting food. The garden needs these organisms to thrive, and you also need these organisms to help build a healthy foundation for you so that you can produce a thriving life. Let's call these little organisms the 'I needs'.

THE DAILY HABIT OF 'I NEED'

Our daily needs are referred to as the things we need to survive such as water, food, and shelter.

What we think we need often gets mixed up with what we only want. Think of value in everything. Everything is useful, there is no clutter.

What value does a cheese pizza or French fry have? It is food, which is a need for survival, right? But would that give you the necessary nutrients to fuel your heart, blood, and muscles for the needed energy for your day? Although my husband says that fat equals flavor in cooking, the type of fat that you consume determines the value that is received.

What about a quinoa salad with black beans, kale, cucumber, avocado, and tomato? Those ingredients are full of both value and quality that lowers one's likelihood of diseases while providing the necessary energy for your daily tasks.[2]

Your clothing is a foundational need that expresses your inmost feelings, yet when you ask yourself what gives value, would a statement necklace keep you warm when it is 40 degrees outside? Of course, a warm versatile jacket would be of more value.

Coco Chanel says, "Before you leave the house, look in the mirror and remove one accessory."

What kind of companions do you associate yourself with? Are those that you surround yourself with uplifting and encouraging? Do they see the good in things and point you towards a better way? Value in companionship comes with high-minded morals, principles, and uplifting behavior.

It is often said, show me your company and I will show you your character.

With thinking of what has value in your life, ask yourself what do you think you need in your life and compare those needs with your wants. You may think that you need to decompress at the end of the day by watching endless hours of TV, but is the need to shut off your frontal lobe competing with what you only truly want?

It is only natural to want to wind down and relax after a long day, yet how you fill that need affects the foundation of your self-care habits and results. A decent replacement for you to still receive the pleasures of relaxation is to go for a walk around the block before entering your home. This will allow for a healthy transition time between your work mind, to your relaxed home mind.

• **What do you think you need in your life?**

ASK YOURSELF

_____

_____

_____

_____

• **How many of those needs are actually wants?**

_____

_____

_____

_____

- **When you want something that is not a need, how can you deal with your wants in a healthy way?**

_____

_____

_____

Knowing with clarity what you need that will provide value to your life is vital to forming a strong foundation when it comes to taking care of yourself. This concept of 'I need' will help you focus on what will truly give you the renewal that self-care provides.

HAVING A STRONG FOUNDATION FOR REGENERATIVE SELF CARE

After knowing and defining your needs while still enjoying your wants, the next step to a healthy foundation for regenerative self-care is living these four simple methods.

1. **Promote sustainability.**
    To have a sustainable self-care routine, you need to protect your mind, body, and soul so that you can survive life occurrences that may throw you a curveball.

When you receive news that your mother has a terminal illness, you lost your job, or your kid comes home with a note from the principal, how would you react? What would be your way of coping?

Without a sustainable self-care routine, you are vulnerable to being worn down, which causes your vital forces to be squandered when life is thrown hard at you. You tend to be more impatient, have low self-esteem, partake in bad habits, and have a poor immune system that is not strong to ward off the bad guys.

To promote a sustainable self-care routine, you need to invest in protecting yourself as a person without any obligations for anyone or anything. This is primarily done with your morning and evening routine.

Guard this time in your day with everything that you have for the sake of your well-being. Carve out time and make it a habit to spend at least 30 minutes or up to two hours investing in building your protection for your mind, body, and soul.

There are many suggestions out there on how to have a thriving morning and evening routine, yet you are unique, so do whatever fills your cup for the day and calms you down before you retire in the evening. Be mindful to choose things that restore, not deplete. This can be a quiet moment to read, stretch and exercise, soak in the bathtub with Epsom salt, or do a hobby that you would not normally have time for in the day.

As a part of your morning and evening routine, practice the habit of 'word setters'. Write words that make you happy, give joy, and allude to a sense of peace. Then ask yourself why do you appreciate these words?

TRY IT!

Example: Care. I love the feeling that I receive when I go out of my way to care for my children and they reciprocate that care in their special way to others.

One action that is depleting to you during your mornings and evenings is the habit of endless scrolling and social media. We are more powerful when we live our lives in a rich way, than staring at a screen, scrolling down the news feed, seeing how many likes we have, and clicking on what is recommended for us. Some algorithms work for our advantages and disadvantages. Most often, the recommended videos or suggestions are an algorithm that is there to think for you and is not there for your advantage. Rather, they are most often not consistent with your goals, your values, and your life.

Search individually for what you want to look for instead of the recommended link so that you can be in control instead of being controlled.

2. Be prepared for unwanted interruptions.

Being mentally prepared for unexpected interruptions or occurrences gives you the power over the situation, not others having power over your reaction.

Unwanted interruptions in your life most often brings about stress. When you are prepared for those unexpected times that cause you stress, it gives you the power to react reasonably. Become aware of what triggers stress in your life, which is anything that alters your normal equilibrium, and do what is necessary to prevent those occurrences or lessen the intensity.

When your body is under stress, your brain releases cortisol, which causes cloudy thinking.[3] So the best way to be prepared for any kind of stress is to recognize that you're not going to be at your best and you should put systems in place so that you can know how to act in the situations which cause you stress or harm.

Going grocery shopping releases a truckload of cortisol in my brain and I end up buying foods that I do not need and forget the items that I went to the store to get. Double that with bringing kids that have not napped or had a meal to eat, and that is a recipe for disaster. So the system that I have in place to lessen my stress and make the shopping experience pleasant for both my kids and myself is to have a list with the items needing to be purchased and my kids with a full belly and rested eyes. This way I do not have to think about what I need to get and can easily grab the items while my kids are happy to go through the grocery store maze excitedly finding each item.

This one day, though, I thought that I could squeeze a run to the grocery store close to suppertime thinking that it will be quick and my kids usually do not act out when I go at other times (forgetting that my system is in place to prevent any outbreaks). This occurrence happened when my kids were younger and my oldest was just learning to potty train and I thought that I could go and come back quick enough in case she had to go.

This grocery shopping experience did not go as well as I was hoping. When we all were in our car seats, myself included, I looked at the clock and was somewhat comforted that I could make it back home for my appointment in time if we leave now. As I am reversing, I hear from the back seat, "Mama, I have to go potty!"

I took a deep breath and weighed the situation. Is it easier to clean up a soiled car seat and clothes and make it back home in time or to trudge back into the grocery store for the restroom? Yes, we all trudged back into the grocery store.

As we were holding hands, one child was pulling me so fast towards the restroom while it seemed as though the other was dragging a ton of bricks. At that moment I was under stress because going to the restroom would now make me late for my appointment. So because of that, my mind was cloudy and I did not even realize that as we were going as fast as we could to get relief for one child, the other had grabbed the produce bags and was pulling one long train across the store aisle before I even noticed.

When I finally turned to see what the heavy pull was, we all stopped and I looked with a gasp. Both of my kids looked at me to see what I would do. Then we all burst out laughing! And let me tell you, all of our attitudes were immediately transformed, for laughter releases endorphins that improve mood and decrease levels of the stress-causing hormones cortisol and adrenaline.[4]

Even though I already had a system in place to not go out shopping with the kids at certain times, I did not heed my preventative preparedness. So, the next best thing that you can do to be prepared is to look on the bright side, which will lighten up the stress and your clouded mind.

3. **Avoid artificial self-care.**
Synthetic self-care is not conducive to a regenerative lifestyle because it creates an imbalance in your mood, mental alertness, and motor performance.

One of the most misused synthetic self-care practices is the use of caffeine. About 89% of US Americans consume caffeine every day, with nearly 75% of children under the age of 18 consuming caffeine every day.[5, 6]

Why is this a synthetic self-care practice?

Caffeine is a stimulant that can aid in alertness, yet it does not provide the alertness and decision-making ability that getting enough sleep can give you.[7] Caffeine also tends to reinforce the development of other unhealthy behaviors while still affecting one's mood, mental alertness, and motor performance.[8]

Creating habits of self-care that supply your body with the appropriate fuel is the best practice for a regenerative lifestyle.

4. Set a timer.

Knowing that there is a reasonable timer that is set on your duties helps your hands work more efficiently.

Time is a very loving, giving, yet very unforgiving thing. Time squandered can never be recovered, yet when you harness the value of time, you can use that power to motivate you to effectively complete each task with diligence.

Setting a timer on your tasks and duties reduces fatigue, long work hours, and exhaustion. Setting a timer and taking an intentional break in between your tasks gives your mind a sufficient amount of time to regenerate and restore your brain's ability to improve depression and your overall well-being.

The sooner you get going setting out to achieve your small success in your daily habits, then the easier it is to get going to reach a lifetime of transformations.

HOW REGENERATIVE SELF-CARE GIVES BACK

The choices you make in your self-care routine directly or indirectly benefit your immediate family, your community, and yourself personally.

Just simply ask yourself, "Are my habits giving back?" When you are watching Netflix hours upon end, what does that do to your physical body, your relationships, your environment, and your personal enrichment goals? Does that give back in any way?

• **Physical Body: what do you do in your self-care routine that gives you peak physical health and quality of life?**

_____

_____

_____

ASK YOURSELF

• **Relational: how do you connect with your family and friends that make your community a better place?**

_____

_____

_____

• **Environment: what are your lifestyle habits when it comes to trash and sustainability? Are you content with your habits?**

_____

_____

_____

• **Personal Enrichment Goals: what lifestyle habits do you do that allow you to reach these goals so that you can give your best?**

_____

_____

_____

• **How can you change your habits that are not regenerative into being ones that benefit society as a whole?**

_____

_____

_____

In the following chapters, we will address specific self-care habits that you do daily, and how each one can be done regeneratively so that they give back to you and your community as a whole.

CHAPTER 4

Mind-Body Connection

"For as he thinks in his heart, so is he."

– KING SOLOMON

According to the Laboratory of Neuro Imaging at the University of Southern California, the average person has about 48.6 thoughts per minute, which adds up to a total of 70,000 thoughts per day.[9] There is no doubt that amidst the thousands of thoughts running through our minds each day and the intensity of life's activities, there is a need for restoration and a renewed mind-body connection. We take a rest every evening, yet even then it seems as though complete rest is not achieved sometimes due to our disquieted mind and body.

The vagus nerve, which is the longest and most complex of the cranial nerves, dominates our parasympathetic nervous system and is responsible for restoring our equilibrium after a stressful event and has been correlated with calming stressful situations.[10]

We are now aware that slow-paced breathing, in a controlled manner, at the right frequency can result in vagal nerve activation, and has been shown to improve anxiety, depression, pain, blood pressure, asthma, irritable bowel syndrome, athletic performance, and cardiovascular health. [11, 12, 13]

Your vagus nerve also has a direct correlation to our Heart Rate Variability (HRV). HRV refers to the time between each heartbeat, and that can vary depending on how you breathe. A healthy heart beats faster when you breathe in and slower when you breathe out.

Check your pulse as you breathe in and out. Did you notice that your pulse was faster when you breathed in and slower when you breathed out? It's pretty neat how your breath affects your pulse, huh!

TRY IT!

Your vagus nerve is so powerful that when you breathe correctly, it can stimulate your prefrontal cortex, which aids in your decision and judgment making while also regulating your heart rate, blood pressure, digestion, and speaking.[14, 15]

BENEFITS OF YOUR MIND BODY CONNECTION

If you would like to partake in the benefits of your mind-body connection, then here are four ways for you to restore your mind-body connection.

1. **Deep breathing.**
    Deep breathing allows you to take a moment to regroup

yourself when things may seem overwhelming.

Our breathing changes during different events, with even our pulse increasing when we inhale.[16] The best practice for deep breathing is to breath 5 or 6 slow controlled breaths per minute, split equally between breathing in and out. The key is to breathe normally, so that you won't hyperventilate.

Do this in the morning to set the tone for the day and in the evening to regroup everything back together.

Want to know if you are breathing correctly? Make sure that your diaphragm is the one doing the work, not your chest. Visualize filling up the lower part of your lungs just above your belly button like a balloon, and then exhaling slowly. You can check yourself by laying flat on the ground and putting your hand on your stomach making sure that it is your stomach that is rising and not your chest. This is going to stimulate your vagus nerve, activate your parasympathetic nervous system, and improve your heart rate variability.

Deep breathing is most beneficial in the fresh outdoor air, and when you do, be sure to take notice of the world around you. Have you stopped recently to listen to a bird's song or noticed the intricate contrast between the green trees and the blue sky?

Once you are used to deep breathing correctly, your body will breathe on its own and you can focus on the beauty around you.[17]

• **What time in the day is best for me to schedule time for deep breathing?**

_____

_____

_____

ASK YOURSELF

• **What location do I see myself getting the best benefits from deep breathing that will also make it easy for me to do it?**

_____

_____

_____

• **How many times a day/week do I wish to practice deep breathing?**

_____

_____

_____

2. Purposeful space.

Every space in our thinking is going to be filled with something. Good or bad.

Each day you are graced with about 70,000 thoughts that pop into your head, which can either be reassuring or stressful. Instead of aimlessly juggling all of your thoughts, channel those ideas into something purposeful and good. If you happen to daydream about a much needed vacation or how to make more readily available healthy food for the underserved, turn those reveries into motivational actions.

• **What is my most recent daydream?**

_____

_____

WRITE IT

• **What do I need to do to make this daydream a reality?**

- How much money is needed?
- How much time needs to be devoted?
- What resources are available?

_____

_____

• **What is the outcome of your daydream that you wish to accomplish?**

_____

_____

_____

_____

ASK YOURSELF

Most likely your environment triggers your thoughts, therefore the first thing to do is change your environment so that your outcome can be changed.

This might look like replacing your snack bowl on your desk or counter that you reach for during stressful moments to your favorite water bottle. It does seem quite unfair that your favorite snack is replaced with just water, but let's give water a chance for one second.

Disruptions in mood and cognitive functioning are brought about by even mild levels of dehydration.[23] For when you are dehydrated, it leads to higher cortisol levels—the stress hormone—which makes it harder to deal with everyday issues. By staying hydrated, you will be less tempted to grab for your snack bowl and be better equipped to deal with everyday problems, therefore making drinking water a win-win.

Mind-Body Connection

- **Does my environment trigger my thoughts of wanting something that is not the best for me?**

_____

_____

_____

_____

- **What can I remove or add to my environment that will motivate, encourage, and promote me to be the best person that I can be?**

_____

_____

_____

_____

3. Rest through hard work.

No, this is not an oxymoron, for it is through hard work on your part that allows you the opportunity to repose.

It has been shown that when cognitive behavioral therapy (CBT) is used, it can change dysfunctions of the nervous system and

63

increase the neural connectivity between your amygdala, which manages your emotions, and your prefrontal cortex, which governs your thinking.[18, 19]

Changing your thought patterns and behavior help you to ultimately cure the root problem. Let's say you want to lower your blood sugar levels, yet you tend to skip breakfast, forget to drink water during the day and only remember to fill up on coffee, you love your pasta, and the last time you exercised was last year.

The root problem is lifestyle habits, yet ultimately it is the negative thought patterns connected to those lifestyle habits that need to be addressed. For each negative thought and action pattern that you partake in, trace it back to the root cause. For example, you skip breakfast. Why? You either ate late the night before, your first 'real' meal was in the evening, or you were snacking during the day just to keep you going.

The thought patterns and behaviors that can cure the root problem is:

• Preparing your breakfast the night before so that it makes it easier to eat in the am if you are in a rush.

• Fill up a mug of water and have it next to your pre-made breakfast so that there is no tendency to forget.

• Replace high carbohydrate meals with high fiber, low glycemic foods such as:[20]

- Vegetables (broccoli, spinach, green peas, beet greens,

brussel sprouts)

- Fruits (apple, pear, peach, nectarine, oranges, berries, dried fruits)

- Beans (kidney, lima, black-eyed, chick peas, lentils)

- Nuts (almonds, pistachios, brazil nuts, soy nuts, walnuts, peanuts)

- Seeds (flaxseed, pumpkin, sesame, sunflower)

- Whole meal bread, multi-grain bread, rye bread

- Bran, oats, whole wheat

• If able, sign up for a 5K with a friend to keep you motivated, otherwise walk at least 30-60 minutes every day.

Will it be hard to prepare your breakfast and get your water ready the night before? At first, maybe, and it may take a while to get used to. Will it be hard eating beans instead of pasta? Most likely if you have hardly eaten beans before. Will it be hard to begin an exercise routine? You may have side cramps and sore muscles, yet it is not impossible.

All of these behaviors take hard work and effort to change to the new desired behavior, yet it is when the hard effort keeps being repeated and engrained, where you can see the results and ultimately take a rest because you are naturally doing what is best for you and it is helping you to thrive.[21]

Your mind is a muscle, and the more that you use it to get the results you desire, the better it performs.

When we change our addictions or any harmful habit, it requires rewiring our brains by growing new connections and neurons.

Psychiatrist John Ratey explains:

"Experiences, thoughts, actions, and emotions actually change the structure of our brains. By viewing the brain as a muscle that can be weakened or strengthened, we can exercise our ability to determine who we become. Indeed, once we understand how the brain develops, we can train our brains for health, vibrancy, and longevity." [22]

Take a moment to think of one problem that you would like to change or fix. Write the problem down, and then trace back to see what are your negative thought patterns or actions that have led to your problem, if any. Then, think of what you can do create your new thoughts or behaviors that can help you in curing your situation.

Problem

_____

_____

Wrong Thought

_____

_____

New Thought

_____

_____

New Behavior

_____

_____

4. Focus not on yourself.

According to the World Happiness Report, people give their time and money to others in return for greater life satisfaction and longer healthier life.[24]

Whether these actions are done intentionally or not, when a charitable donation is given or a voluntary good deed is performed, it activates the reward center of our brains.[25] Positive reinforcement and its benefits naturally occur when we put our energies to focus on those around us.

A few ways to focus on others:

• Donate blood. If you are in healthy perimeters for being a prospective blood donor, take the time to save a life today.

• Fill up. Where able, fill up someone's gas tank, pay for the tables bill next to you at the restaurant, fill up someone's parking meter that is about to expire.

• Volunteer. Contact local charities such as food banks, churches, and even pet adoption centers for any needs that may be present.

• Mow a neighbors lawn.

• Contribute Financially. Local charities and if able, giving means for clothing or food essentials for those who are in need will go a long way.

• **What are some other ways that I can focus on others that resonate with who I am?**

WRITE IT

_____

_____

_____

Each new day gives you new thoughts and new events. The power lies in you to choose what kind of thoughts will fill your mind and what new event you will act out.

As each day is granted to you, remember to breathe mindfully so that you can be calm, work so that you may rest, fill all empty spaces with good, and pay attention to others around you and fill their lives with the joy that you can give either through your time, actions, or your generous monetary gifts.

CHAPTER 5

Locally Grown

*"Good nutrition creates health in all areas of our existence.
All parts are interconnected."*

– T. COLLIN CAMPBELL

Before we got married, my husband said that he would cook for me for the rest of my life. He had me when he said that, because I for sure needed someone in my life that I didn't have to win his heart over with my cooking.

I just need to remind him of this more often because I somehow got the end of the deal that I am cooking most of the time now. Thankfully, I can cook more than boiling water when we first met. But when my husband does cook, he finds the most amazing chefs around the world and he then makes his rendition of that food.

It is through this experience that it has shown me how produce tastes so much better when we eat locally and in season, rather than in bulk with no consideration as to where the food came from or if it was picked in the time of its season.

My husband would bring fresh produce home that would fill the entire home with its incredible aroma. It would lure me into the kitchen and I would want to eat it right then and there. Even more so, I couldn't wait to eat it when he plated in front of me the delicious food that he had made. To this day, my favorite thing to have in my fridge is locally grown, in season fresh herbs and produce.

Try cooking a dish that is locally grown and in season.

I want to share with you four of our favorite dishes that my husband makes from fresh herbs. There is a recipe to try for each of the four seasons. Enjoy!

Once we began to experience and taste the difference between fresh, in season produce compared to buying produce in bulk all year round with no thought of when the item is actually in season, our lives changed for the better. We then began to be conscious of where we would buy our produce, when we would buy, and what type of produce we would buy.

FOOD CAN ALSO BE A HIJACKER

Let me tell you, though, when I was growing up and not until the moment when my husband and I began buying locally and cooking in season that I did not make the best of choices in my eating habits. There was no connection in my brain between the choices of food that I ate to the effect that it was having upon my body, the local community, and the effect of harming the environment.

My friends and I would go surfing while eating a whole box of Dunkin Donuts. Most of my food items of choice would not be fresh and in season, but they would be highly processed, loaded with sugar, and contain a low nutritional value. Mostly packaged foods and fast food.

In most cases, food is a weak spot. For when you eat something enjoyable, whether healthy or not, our brains experience a triggered excitement from the dopamine release during the experience of the activity. Foods that are highly processed, fried, and contain a high sugar content actuality hijack the true experience of a healthy dopamine rush that eating fresh local produce can give.

Growing up I would not have made the connection, but I will never forget the McDonald's sign that I saw several years ago which said:

Cravings, take the wheel.

Next to those words, it had a delicious looking picture of a McChicken Sandwich and French fries. Many times I can remember my Dad looking at a road sign similar to that one and he would end up pulling over and buying food from that fast food place because he said it looked good.

Blown away by the boldness to show the vulnerability that one has when it comes to food and the effect that food has to bypass the capability of our mind to make an educated decision when our mind is hijacked with the distorted dopamine rush from unhealthy foods, that now made me sick to my stomach.

Food brings pleasure while also fueling our daily needs, yet our culture in America has made it not common to think that fresh food is better for our health and environment. This is where the power lies in you to go against the grain and choose what kind of food that you consume that will give you the ability to think clearly from a healthy dopamine rush, rather than being hijacked by your unhealthy food choices.

The best ways to take care of your mind and body where you can trigger that dopamine rush healthily is to:

1. **Eat foods rich in Tyrosine.**
   Enzymes in your body help turn Tyrosine into dopamine, therefore making it important to have an adequate amount of it.

Tyrosine is an amino acid that is a part of the building blocks of protein. The best form to ingest tyrosine is through foods such as soybeans, almonds, bananas, avocados, beans, pumpkin and sesame seeds, wild rice, oats, and wheat.[26]

While I do know that there are meat sources that are rich in tyrosine also, I have only listed plant-based references for the fact that plants have a lower carbon footprint, are more ethical, and offer greater nutritional value. When considering any food item in concerning regeneration, be mindful of how big their feet are.

2. Improve gut health.

Certain bacteria in your gut are capable of producing dopamine and reducing symptoms of anxiety and depression.[27]

Probiotics improve your gut health and increase dopamine levels by consuming these foods: yogurt, kefir, Sauerkraut, tempeh, kimchi, miso, kombucha, pickles, natto, and probiotic supplements.

Most of these food items mentioned to improve your gut health can be eaten all year round since they are fermented.

3. High fiber foods.

Plant foods provide the greatest amount of fiber and give you a sense of being full, therefore giving your mind a healthy dopamine rush and satisfaction.

Foods that are high in fiber are raspberries, pear, apple, green peas, broccoli, beets, barley, quinoa, brown rice, split peas, lentils, black beans, and chia seed.

Wherever you are in the world, the time that these foods are grown that are mentioned above may vary due to the environment and weather. Being mindful of knowing when the foods you consume are in season will trigger the natural regenerative cycle in food.

Sustainable eating will give you the empowerment to make

changes within your realm, which in turn will give you the confidence and satisfaction knowing that you are taking hold of the power that lies in you to make a change for the better.

WHAT TYPE OF PRODUCE IS BEST

Organic or Biodynamic. These words may be the first ones that come to mind when you think of sustainable eating, but there is one lifestyle choice of eating that I believe surpasses organic and biodynamic. Locally Grown. Let me explain. When you are at the grocery store looking at different types of foods and produce, you may notice different words that are used to describe the food item such as whole grain and natural. These labels may sound healthy and seem to be a good choice, but in actuality, these terms are not specific nor do they require any regulations.

The term organic, on the other hand, is certified by the United States Department of Agriculture (USDA), and it means something very specific. Organic means that the produce or food item was grown without any synthetic pesticides and fertilizers that don't include any genetically modified organisms.[28]

Organic animal products mean that they are grown without any antibiotics or growth hormones, but the focus on organic and locally grown in this nutrition portion is about fresh produce.

The purpose for farmers to use pesticides and fertilizers on their crops is to provide a large amount of food to feed the high demand for food from the 329 million people living in the United States, which continues to grow. While having enough food to feed the growing population is a good thing, the negative payoff is that our environment and personal health take a hit.

Fertilizers and pesticides are made from fossil fuels, which means they release greenhouse gases into the environment.[29] Not only are workers who daily handle these fertilizers and pesticides being exposed to chlorpyrifos and glyphosate, which take a severe health risk such as dermatological, gastrointestinal, neurological, carcinogenic, respiratory, reproductive, and endocrine effects, but the extra fertilizer that is sprayed on the crops ends up running into our lakes, rivers and eventually into the ocean.[30]

When these fertilizers and pesticides end up in the ocean, it removes the necessary oxygen that is needed to support any marine life, therefore damaging the eco system.[31, 32]

Since organic farming methods do not use synthetic fertilizers and pesticides, it has a three-fold positive effect:

1. Organic farming protects the farm worker from harmful exposure.
2. Organic farming protects the environment.
3. Organic farming protects us from not being at less risk for consuming pesticide residues from the food that we eat.

While organic farming is good at protecting the farm worker, the environment, providing fewer pesticides in our food, and is the standard for the production of organic food, organic farming does not focus on rebuilding or regenerating the soil.

Regenerative farming supports the farmers and ranchers by using everything that interacts in the environment such as the soil, water, plants, animals, and even us humans. This regenerative process provides cleaner air, water, food, and an overall healthier environment for us to live in, therefore meaning that everything works together with a focus on the outcome. An outcome that actually improves the health of the soil and land.

It is this concept of regenerative farming that is woven into a lifestyle of regenerative self-care. The principle is to focus on the outcome of a healthier you by using your unique and natural temperament, your resources around you, and your life dynamics to provide a strong life.

Just like working with nature is complex, so is working with yourself. If a good practice is applied at the wrong time or not in alignment with who you are, it can hurt you instead of helping to restore and satisfy.

Regenerative self-care is not about *practicing* self-care, but about *living* self-care.

So, do you want to know where to buy your produce? Ok, let's get back to the good stuff. Food.

WHERE TO BUY YOUR PRODUCE

This is where locally grown comes in. Most supermarkets label their foods and tell you where it is grown, usually from within your state. While a local Farmer's Market allows you to not only get locally grown foods within a 100-mile radius or smaller, but it gives you the power to support your local farmers.

A lot of local farmers are not certified organic because they may not be big enough to pay the fee for the "Organic" title, but they tend to already use fewer chemicals than the standard non-organic farms. The Environmental Working Group (EWG) provides a quick guide for produce that contains high and low pesticides for those concerned about which ones to purchase organic or not.[33]

Knowing where our food was grown improves the amount of nutrients that we consume. For when produce has to be picked unripe and shipped and stored over a long period of time, the nutrients and vitamins that are found in those fruits and vegetables are lost.

I love my bananas and I always joke that I want to plant a banana tree in my back yard, but when you purchase them from another country out of season, they are typically picked green and then synthetically ripened with ethylene gas for the population demand.

Not only does produce that is bought locally and personally picked from the tree typically taste better and provide a higher nutritional content, but it also traveled a shorter distance from the garden to your mouth, therefore having a smaller carbon footprint.

Our family is privileged to have a local farmer's market that is open all year round where we can have access to sustainable seasonal produce. This allows us to talk to the local farmers and ask them how their crops were grown, which makes it more personal.

When the weather is nice, we walk there as a family and have the kids choose items that they enjoy. My daughter looks forward to the strawberries in the summer and choosing special flowers for our kitchen table.

The USDA provides a search for local Farmer's Markets in your area, so take a look at which ones are close by you and enjoy the benefits of local produce!

It is also our family tradition to every season go picking at a local farm for produce that is in season. This helps us understand the work that is involved in bringing the produce to the grocery store for us to purchase, while also enjoying firsthand the deliciousness that comes from a freshly picked strawberry, blackberry, apricot, peach, nectarine, tomato, apple, cucumber, and pumpkin.

Whenever possible, buy locally grown. Even better, plant a small garden where you can witness and enjoy the fruits of your labor. The results from the foods that you consume from local farming will not only be better for you, better for your environment, but it will also improve your mental outlook when you partake in being a part of this sustainability by gardening your foods.[34]

WHEN TO BUY YOUR PRODUCE

Most of the western world has provided ease in shopping for produce. This has made it super convenient to buy produce at your leisure any time of the year. The downside with this is there is a temptation to lose connection with your food, the farmer, and the benefits of eating seasonally.

In America, it is harder to tell which foods are in season because the grocery store has the same staple produce each and every day no matter what season it is, but if you were to go to another country you would see street corners filled with exuberant amounts of fresh produce that change with the seasons as the local's way of making money.

There was a location in South Africa where grocery stores were not common, yet there were these really neat shops that were a colonial-style farmers market where the locals would sell hand made sustainable clothing and have these impressive bakeries with freshly baked bread, local preserves, and scrumptious fresh and local cheeses. I do not typically consume dairy products, but these cheeses smelled so fresh and delicious that I had to try them on the freshly baked bread. I still remember that dopamine rush.

In Fiji, the local farmer's market was bigger than I have ever seen. Rows and rows of fresh greens, kinds that I have never seen or heard of before. Instead of grocery carts, we used wheelbarrows. For myself, my husband, and two of our friends, we filled two huge wheelbarrows with every color of produce you can think of. And we ate every bit of that fresh produce. The flavor that the fresh produce provided as we ate it, was beyond comparable.

A very traditional Fijian meal is cooked in a lovo, an underground oven, where each food item is wrapped in banana leaves and then slowly baked for hours. These foods like taro, cassava, wild yams, turnips, and proteins, get a rich smoky flavor. Fijians are very resourceful, they don't just use the taro root, they also stew the leaves. For a lighter flavor, local tree ferns (Otta) are boiled and then seasoned with onions, tomato, and fresh coconut milk. All of these flavors come together in such a taste of Polynesian paradise, all from local ingredients.

The produce there is not like what you would expect in America, like romaine lettuce, or cherry tomatoes. Instead of wishing for something that they didn't have locally, the Fijians cook and prepare what is naturally grown in their environment and make it delicious.

The Philippines would take advantage of the tropical weather and have mango and banana trees in their tiny backyard porches. In every home that I went to, I was amazed that each one had a mango tree and sometimes a banana tree in their tiny little backyard. There was a sense of pleasure being able to pick and eat a juicy mango straight from the tree with less than one foot of carbon footprint. Street corners would be bustling with local fresh produce for the people in the village to buy. Since most homes did not have any refrigerator, each day fresh produce would be bought for their family.

These memories and experiences that I have been blessed to live and enjoy helped me to understand that where you are in the world affects how you buy and consume your produce. These places that I had the privilege to be immersed in their lifestyle already practiced living locally and in season daily. This was their life.

For those who live in the Western World, where eating locally and in season may not come as naturally because of the convenience at hand, here are four ways to help you begin being more aware of the power that your choices have to make a difference in the world.

1. Grow your own food.

Even if you do not have a green thumb, planting a simple indoor herb garden could dramatically change the value of the food that you consume.

2. Buy from a local farmer's market.

If you are privileged to have a farmers market in your local community, take advantage of that and get to know the farmers that are providing the food that you are buying from.

In my local farmer's market, I would go to this one farmer every time for our strawberries. I would talk to them, get to know them personally, and find out their farming practices during each visit.

This one time, instead of going there first, I went at the end of our trip when my cash supply was low without me realizing it. Because I had already built a friendship with the farmers they let me take the strawberries and said to pay them the next time I came. I did pay, plus extra for their kindness. But when would you get an experience like that at a grocery store?

I used to work at a supermarket and I would do my best to connect with the customers that would come consistently. So, yes, you can build relationships with your local grocery store workers, but never had I experienced such a close connection with the individual who grew the food that I would be eating.

3. **Purchase a subscription to a Community Supported Agriculture produce delivery box.**

If you are uncertain what produce is in season and do not have a local farmers market, you can support a local Community Supported Agriculture (CSA) produce delivery box. They deliver to your door fresh picked produce of your choice from their local farm. We have tried different local ones in our area like Farm Fresh To You, but that may not be available in your local area, so search which CSA boxes are local.

4. **Buy locally grown produce in your grocery store.**

You can still consume foods that are in season and grown locally in your grocery store supermarket. It is becoming more common to find a section in the produce area where it is just for locally grown produce. I have also seen at certain grocery stores tags that say which farm the produce was grown on and how far it traveled to get to the grocery store.

What is your goal for the next two weeks? Instead of having a set menu and then trying to find your produce, reverse it. Find what is available and then shape your meals accordingly.

If you don't eat locally for the most part, start small. Start with 1-2 meals per week that are mostly made from locally grown produce. Once that becomes a habit, then aim for half of your meals. Once you have mastered 50% of your meals locally grown, then plan to prepare as close to the majority of your food consumption from locally grown produce.

TRY IT!

• **What places are around your area that you can go and purchase locally grown produce?**

_____

_____

_____

_____

ASK YOURSELF

• **What local produce did you discover available that you did not know before?**

_____

_____

_____

• **What meals can you prepare with that local produce?**

_____

_____

_____

We make a lot of food choices in one single day, so why not use the power that lies in you to make regenerative eating habits by knowing where your food comes from, supporting local farmers, and cooking home meals more often.

CHAPTER 6

Personal Care Products

"Take care of your body. It's the only place you have to live."

– Jim Rohn

There is a family of chemicals termed as 'forever chemicals'. Some of the few ways that we come in contact with these forever chemicals is through the water we drink, the cookware we use, and the clothes that we wear. The bad thing about this 'family' is that they are harmful to our bodies and to the environment that we call our home.

Similar to these forever chemicals are certain hormone-altering chemicals that can be found in our cosmetics, personal care products, and cleaning products. These chemicals alter our hormones by disrupting our endocrine system, therefore calling them endocrine disruptors.

Our endocrine system is a network of hormone-producing glands and is crucial for your development, metabolism, sleep, and reproduction. When this system is altered, it can cause fatigue, constipation or stomach upset, dehydration, abnormal bone growth, and depression.[35]

CHECK YOUR INGREDIENTS

It's important to check your personal care product labels. Not only should you check your grocery food labels, but also your lotions, mascara, foundations, shampoos, and nail polish are just as important.

The main endocrine disruptor ingredients that are found in personal care products are phthalates and glycol ethers. Since a lot of studies has been done on these chemicals and there has been a greater awareness of the great harm of these ingredients in common personal care products and cleaning supplies, there is seen a greater demand for phthalate and sulfate-free products.

A few of the most common phthalates and glycol ethers to look out for are:[36, 37]

PHTHALATES

Name	Acronym
Diisononyl phthalate	DINP
Dimethyl phthalate	DMP
Diethyl phthalate	DEP
Butyl benzyl phthalate	BBP
Diisodecyl phthalate	DIDP
Di(2-ethylhexyl) phthalate	DEHP, DOP

GLYCOL ETHERS

NAME

Acetic Acid

2-Phenoxyethyl Ester

Ethane

Butane

Stearate

Stearic Acid

Polyethylene

You don't have to be a nerd like me and read every ingredient and research where it comes from and what it does to your mind, body, and the environment. Yet, you can use this powerful tool that the Environmental Working Group (EWG) has put together, called the Skin Deep Cosmetic Database, and use it to search your favorite personal care product to see how the ingredients affect you and the environment. Consider this your cheat sheet!

Pick one personal care product. What are the ingredients in it? Are any of those ingredients harmful? If your product scores high on the Environmental Working Group Skin Deep Cosmetic Database, what are some other possible healthier replacement products?

MAKE YOUR OWN

For those of you who love making things with your hands and don't mind experimenting with new things, then an option for you to make sure your personal care products and cleaning supplies are free of unwanted chemicals is to make them yourself.

You know how it is said, that if you're going to quit, you might as well quit cold turkey. Well, I did that with all of my personal care products and my hair and skin was in chaos! It was as if my hair didn't know how to hold a curl and my skin was breaking out like I was a teenager. This was all happening because my body was going through a chemical detox. This went on for several weeks and I was beginning to wonder if this is natural and thought to go back to the products that I was used to using.

I am glad that I didn't, because shortly after my debating stage, I began to notice a difference. I noticed that my hair went back to its normal wave, but this time with more volume, and my skin began to feel a whole lot younger without all the breakouts.

When I began to make my homemade personal care items, I threw away all of my shampoos, body wash, makeup, cleaning supplies, and anything that contained any harmful chemical. Then I began to make, one by one: lotion, face wash and moisturizer, body wash, shampoo, conditioner, deodorant, hand soap, makeup, dishwasher soap, and other household cleaning products.

Thankfully my husband did not freak out too much when he saw unused products in the trashcan and he was such a good sport in trying new things.

Now, the homemade items that I make are few because I have found a company that provides a portion of items that I am happy to use.[38]

You can explore the Internet and find fun personal care products and cleaning supplies to make or you can purchase an increasing amount of cleaner personal care products at your local store.

Make your own hand soap, shampoo, and lotion. See how you feel after you use it. If you like it so much, make some extra and give it as a gift to others. Below is my favorite eye cream that I make and I want to share it with you. It's super simple and easy. Have fun!

TRY IT!

COCONUT OIL EYE CREAM

½ cup room temperature coconut oil

1 teaspoon Vitamin E oil

2 to 3 drops Rose essential oil

Start with room temperature coconut oil in a small bowl. You want to have the coconut oil a paste-like consistency. If it's too warm it will be runny, and if it's too cold it will set up as a solid.

Add the Vitamin E oil and Rose essential oil and mix to combine.

Apply to clean face morning and evening.

Coconut oil hydrates and soothes, Vitamin E oil helps to replenish and restore collagen, while Rose essential oil encourages your skin to retain moisture.

USE YOUR VOICE

Self-education is the best thing that we can do for ourselves. When we become educated with what is in the products that we consume and purchase, we are then empowered to make changes that are better for the environment and us.

I have to admit one thing. I have not worn one piece of makeup for a while now, nor have I used any commercial brand personal care product such as lotions or hair products for the last several years. The products that I use either do not contain any of the endocrine disruptor ingredients or I choose to make my own. So why in the world would it matter to me what is in cosmetic or personal care products?

There are three reasons.

1. Knowledge and education is power.

It is this same knowledge that has led me on the journey from using the cheapest cosmetics with the highest chemical and endocrine disruptor ingredients, to purchasing cosmetics that score decently on the EWG cosmetic database, to ultimately removing all cosmetic products and confidently wearing my God given skin.

2. Conviction is power.

The second reason is when you are convicted about something, you have the voice and power as an individual to encourage the cosmetic industry to generate healthier cosmetics and personal care products so that individuals that may not know of the associations between the use of these personal care products and the links to cancer and endocrine disruptor associations can use them without the negative ramifications.

3. Better future.

Ultimately, it matters to me what is in cosmetic and personal care products because of my children. Years down the road, if they so choose to purchase and wear cosmetic products, I want to know that I did everything in my power to make available to them healthier cosmetic and personal care options.

Use your knowledge to exercise your right to make a change and strive for safer cosmetics. You can use the power that lies in you to contact your Congress representative to encourage them to review and remove unsafe and dangerous cosmetic and personal care product ingredients that are associated with cancers and endocrine disruptors. Your voice does make a difference!

CHAPTER 7

The Not So Typical Exercise

*"Those who contemplate the beauty of the earth find
reserves of strength that will endure as long as life lasts."*

– RACHEL CARSON

I would tell of how three girls would run up the creek splishing and splashing while watching the water level rise taller and taller, climb up the creek walls to pass over a tree branch in the way, squeeze through a portion of a storm drain, and come home soaking wet laughing with joy to only get out and do it all over again.

Then they would say, please just one more story.

Then I would tell of how three girls would run through corn stalks playing hide and seek, climb up trees to see what was beyond, and how a favorite spot of respite was under a humble fig tree.

Then the sleepy eyes would drift off to sleep.

As I headed to my room to do my evening routine, I stopped dead in my tracks and asked myself, "Am I providing my kids this same opportunity to experience these kinds of adventures in the beauty of the earth as I was given when I was a little girl?"

Even though I would take my kids to the beach with every opportunity (every day if it was my choice), let them play and explore outside rain or shine, and plant and grow a little garden plot, I still felt like they could experience more from the beautiful earth that we are blessed with to enjoy.

ANXIETY OF KIDS TODAY

Now more than ever kids are spending too much time indoors, and if they do go outside, there are limitations to their imaginations and their play is structured. We as adults are in the same boat.

Since the Covid-19 pandemic, individuals aged 15 and older spent an average of 2.1 more hours at home in 2020 than in 2019, with a total of 9.7 hours during their waking hours. To go a little deeper, individuals aged 15 and older spent an average of 1.7 hours more per day alone in 2020 than in 2019. And even deeper, individuals aged 55 and older averaged about 8 hours or more per day alone during their waking hours in 2020 than in 2019.[39]

These are scary numbers that have all been attributed to the increase in depression, anxiety, and loneliness in these recent years.

ANXIETY OF ADULTS TODAY

The percentage of adults with recent symptoms of anxiety and depression has increased by 5.1 % in 2021. The worst part of this all is the increase of unmet mental health care, which has increased from 9.2% to 11.7%.[40]

Is there a connection between spending more of our time indoors and not exploring the earth as before to the increase of poor mental health in individuals today?

BEING IN NATURE AS YOUR DOCTOR

Experiences in nature can relieve even the slightest strain on everyday stresses.[41] Nature is most often overlooked as the cheapest, simplest, and most rewarding healing balm for anyone's emotional hardships.

People who are exposed to urban environments are forced to use their attention to overcome the effects of constant stimulation. While on the contrary, when people are in a natural environment, such as being outside in nature, they elicit feelings of pleasure.[42]

Being in nature can be your doctor in four main ways:

1. **Lessens anxiety and stress.**

Even those in the hospital have been shown to heal faster and experience less pain and stress when they have a window to look out at compared to those who do not. Resting in nature naturally reduces your cortisol and adrenaline levels.

2. Boosts creativity and alertness.

The best natural method to boost your sluggish body and mind is to take a break in nature. If you aren't able to go outside or you have no access to a green tree, then go outside and look at a picture of nature.

3. Improves your immune system.

Being outside in the sun naturally gives your body Vitamin D, which helps build your immune system and helps your body absorb calcium. Even if you live in a place that rains the majority of the time or the days are super short, just being close to plants outside will help you feel better.

In Japan, there is a common forest bathing that is called Shinrinyoku, or natural aromatherapy. What happens during these quick trips to the forest is that while you are relaxing, the plants release something that is called phytoncides, or wood essential oils of the tree that are antimicrobial volatile organic compounds.

These forest bathings stimulate your natural killer activity, which helps destroy tumor cells and infected cells.[43]

4. Increases your self-esteem.

Just five minutes each day of outdoor activity could improve the way you think about yourself. Now that doesn't mean you set a timer to go back inside after five minutes, but it also doesn't mean that you have to intensely work up a sweat in those five minutes.[44]

The time when you are outdoors could be a leisure walk, working in your garden, or even chasing a squirrel. The benefits are there no matter what you do, as long as you are outside.

BENEFITS OF EXERCISING IN NATURE

I exercise every day, all day. From the moment that my eyes open till the weight of my eyelids close in retirement at night, I am running. By how much I run in the day, I might as well be a professional marathon runner.

It's too bad that this entire running that I do is not physical running, but unfortunately, it is done by my thoughts.

Does this sound like you?

The expression "your thoughts are running a mile a minute" is no joke. Society has made it the commonplace for the minute you wake up, you are needing to think of food for the family, checklists to be done, meetings to attend, email and phone calls, and deadlines. To top it off, any quiet time that you do have your mind is continually rehashing over and over the things that have happened and what should have been done or still needs to be done.

Now let's think of the flip side. You now have to transition your work to a home station, make sure that your children are connecting to their teachers online without being distracted with everything else when school is closed, and wondering what you will use for your bathroom needs when your last square of toilet paper is used.

When this anxiety tends to lurk around you, it may cause a cloudy mind that is incapable of even accomplishing any of the daily tasks pulling at us each day, therefore resulting in mental and physical burnout.[45]

Although our minds are amazing in themselves, there is still the capability of being at risk for anxiety and depression associated with our running thoughts. The only way to combat our raging thoughts that constantly are at play is to take time.

Take time running.

Sometimes the best cure for something is to tackle it with its own medicine, and this is precisely what running does for our minds.

The amazing thing about running is that the benefits of running outside have greater results than if you were to run indoors on a treadmill. Running outside gives you more energy, and lessens your tension, anger, and depression compared to when you run indoors.[46]

Both runners and non-runners alike are affected the same by depression and anxiety, but what makes the difference between the two is the outcome.

Scott Douglas explains in *Running is My Therapy*, that those who engage in running exercise can process their anxiety and depression in a way that allows their minds to think through their internal 'running' dialogue and resulting actions.

Runners naturally tend to incorporate Cognitive Behavioral Therapy (CBT) during their running times as a way of motivation and competition.[47] The significant thing is that by practicing CBT while running, you are empowering yourself to do the same in your everyday interactions. Research is now showing that individuals who begin using CBT change one's brain that is affected by anxiety.[48]

Now, let's be honest that when your thighs feel like burning firecrackers, your shins are as tight as a braces band, and you have a side cramp that feels like 10,000 knives are stabbing you with more intensity during each breath, the last thing that you desire to do is to continue that run. If this happens to be you also, do not give up hope, for the honeymoon stage will come shortly.

Persistence has shown that those who run consistently have approximately twice the effect of improved mood, vigor, and decreased fatigue than those who do not run or exercise.[49] The key here is to not push yourself so hard that every time you have side cramps or burning thighs, but to get your heart rate at 70-85 percent of your age-adjusted maximum heart rate. When this is done, you not only experience the endorphins from a challenging run or workout, but it can trigger endocannabinoids, which makes a bigger impact on your brain.[50]

Exercise intervention on mental health can be a powerful intervention for clinical depression.[51] Evidence suggests that physical exercise plays a role in building resilience to stress.[52]

Exercise and running have an internal feel good not only for our thoughts, but also for our outlook. We are empowered when we make the effort to go outside, run and push ourselves to conquer the present situation. The amazing thing is when we have success on the toughest day, but continue to defeat each run, then getting out the door the next time is so much easier. The more that we do this while running, the more habitual it will become to implement these habits into our everyday lives of our work and home life.

It takes strength and determination to see the difficulty ahead and go through them with sound bodies and strong minds. It is strong minds that can wrestle with hard problems and conquer them.

Whether it is pushing yourself past running cramps, taking a deep breath when someone cuts you off while driving, or calmly working out a dispute with another individual, empowerment lies at each of our fingertips.

If you are capable of running, tie up your laces and begin introducing into your lifestyle moderate-intensity activity throughout the day and as much running as able. And even you are unable to run, there are other exercises to consider such as swimming, tennis, biking, and even household duties such as raking leaves and intense floor mopping.[53]

As with all exercise routines, moderate physical activity is safe for most people, but it is recommended to check with your doctor before starting any exercise routine.

BACK TO NATURE AN ESSENTIAL

If exercising indoors is all that you can do at this moment, keep it up. Any type of exercise is beneficial for your well-being. For those who can go outside and touch the earth, breathe in the fresh air, and explore without limits, you will experience first hand the benefits of exercise in the great outdoors.

During the 1870s, the Quaker's Friends Hospital in Pennsylvania used natural landscape on acres of land as a part of treating those with mental illness. Then, after WW11, Carl Menninger led a horticulture therapy movement in the Veterans Administration Hospital as a means of using gardening to benefit those with chronic illnesses.

Spending time outdoors has been proven to improve your overall health, well-being, mental health, while also reducing your stress.

So why not take advantage of that?

How can you incorporate being outside into your daily routine?

• **What are things that I can do outside?**

_____

_____

_____

• **How can I change my habits to be more in nature? Are there things that I normally do inside that I can easily do outside as well?**

_____

_____

_____

_____

• **Who can I ask to go outside with me?**

_____

_____

_____

_____

HOW TO TAKE ACTION

Use nature as a means to strengthen family bonds. My fondest memories have always been associated with being outdoors, and I desire to have memories like that for my children as well.

Use your time in nature to reconnect without any technology, and disengage from other distractions so that you can focus on those with you and what is around you.

Our first family camping trip when I was little was in Zion National Forest. It was forecasted to rain, but we still went with a couple of other families who had travel trailers. We did not have the luxury of camping in style, but in my opinion, we had the best. A humble tent. We enjoyed the beauty of the Park and after our hike, we settled into our camp for the night.

We were staying a couple of nights and the first night there, it poured and poured. Our tent did not hold out the rain and everyone but myself had wet sleeping bags. My Dad said we were not staying another night in a wet sleeping bag, so we said goodbye to our friends and went home early from our family camping trip.

Even though it may have been a negative experience with being wet and cold, all of that is only remembered when it is brought up. What stuck with me all these years was the enjoyable time that we had with our friends, drinking hot cocoa, playing games, and the funny memory of everyone in our tent being wet except me.

When you create memories with your loved ones outside, there is something powerful that bonds you closer together. You get your exercise while setting up a tent, walking up a trail, kayaking down a river, or running from a rattlesnake, all the while building lasting memories that can be told to generations to come.

Can you say that your kids have had the same experience as you did when you were young? And if you did not have this experience, can you say that your offspring has opportunities that you may not have had? If you answer no to this simple question, sincerely ask yourself how you can make any changes in your life so that future generations can tell the same stories to their children.

The power lies in you to change the statistics to a decrease instead of an increase and build those priceless bonds with those whom you love.

CHAPTER 8

Social Connection

"We cannot live only for ourselves. A thousand fibers connect us with our fellow men; and among those fibers, as sympathetic threats, our actions run as causes, and they come back to us as effects."

– HERMAN MELVILLE

Self-care is commonly the thought that you have to think about yourself, and thinking of yourself is a good thing. Taking care of yourself and making sure that your needs are met is extremely important in your well-being, yet it is when you think of others by your actions and thoughts that you are then taking care of yourself. True regenerative self-care gives, while also giving back.

IS THINKING ABOUT WHAT IS BEST FOR ME IDEAL?

A doctor, a lawyer, a little boy, and a priest were out for a Sunday afternoon flight on a small private plane. Suddenly, the plane developed engine trouble. Despite the best efforts of the pilot, the plane started to go down. Finally, the pilot grabbed a parachute and yelled to the passengers that they better jump, and he bailed out.

Unfortunately, only three parachutes were remaining.

The doctor grabbed one and said "I'm a doctor, I save lives, so I must live," and jumped out.

The lawyer then said, "I'm a lawyer and lawyers are the smartest people in the world. I deserve to live." He also grabbed a parachute and jumped.

The priest looked at the little boy and said, "My son, I've lived a long and full life. You are young and have your whole life ahead of you. Take the last parachute and live in peace."

The little boy handed the parachute back to the priest and said, "Not to worry, the smartest man in the world just took off with my backpack."

The point of this story is that thinking about what is best for you does not always prove to be the most suitable choice, with a tendency to justify our acts. But do our acts benefit others and take into account what their needs are?

SOMETIMES SELFISHNESS SEEMS THE BEST WAY

Being self-interested is often considered a benefit. For if you are to give your time and money for others then there is less time and money for yourself.[54] What is so wrong with being selfish if it is a benefit to oneself? Let's look at selfishness from three different perspectives.

1. Bad selfishness.

What makes selfishness bad is when one or more persons lose something or is hurt in the process of another person's gain or benefit. Selfishness from this perspective tends to stem from the absence of certain emotions or the presence of others that may signal selfish motivations. [55]

While the gain or benefit for the selfish person may be temporary, the consequences outweigh temporary gains. This can be seen in selfish acts such as assault and fraud, which can result in fines and incarceration.

2. Natural selfishness.

Taking care of you would fit into this category of selfishness. Taking the time to prepare a healthy meal, ensuring that you get the proper amount of sleep, drinking adequate amounts of water, and brushing your teeth would be considered acts that neither take away from someone else's well being nor adds to it, unless that healthy cooked meal is for them also.

3. Good Selfishness.

This perspective of selfishness benefits both you and other people. This can be going on a bike ride with someone and exchanging laughter while building lasting memories. Buying a house is considered another aspect of good selfishness because even though the seller lost the house, he gained monetary value. And while the buyer lost money, he gained a house.

COMMUNAL GOALS AND VALUES BENEFIT ALL INDIVIDUALS INVOLVED

The concept of good selfishness was studied amongst 5th graders when they were asked which method of goal teaching was more valued.

Competitive: "the challenge of seeing who is best"

Individualistic: "enjoying solving problems all on her or his efforts"

Communal: "it's a good idea to help each other learn" and "you can learn a lot of important things from each other"

The results showed that the 5th-grade students preferred communal classroom goals.[56]

When we have this concept of learning from each other and valuing each other's insights, it breaks down the barriers between what occupation you are in, which neighborhood you live in, and even what family you are a part of.

When one exhibits selfishness that is at the expense of other people, it can break any supportive connection with the other individuals.

Yet, when you display otherish motivation or caring for the needs of others, it has the effect to build supportive connections with others.[57] For seeing value in another person's life and yours, it depends crucially upon creating, maintaining, and strengthening the social bonds with each other, no matter our race, socioeconomic status, or beliefs.

HOW TO OBTAIN GENUINE UNSELFISHNESS

To find value in another person when it is so much easier to put your needs and desires above the other means to love unselfishly and aspire to do what is best for them without any motivation for reciprocation.

This is true unselfishness that exceeds good selfishness or communal values. The power lies in you to choose to practice unselfishness to those whom you are connected with either by family, friends, or social acquaintances.

The best part is that these altruistic acts and desires can be obtained by stimulating your prefrontal cortex. The best ways to do this is by:

1. **Breathing.**

Slow-paced breathing, in a controlled manner, at the right frequency can result in vagal nerve activation.[58] When the vagus nerve is activated it stimulates your prefrontal cortex, which aids in your decision and judgment making.[59] The vagus nerve stimulation and the triggering of the prefrontal cortex bring about a more generous attitude and unselfish behavior.[60]

2. **Being Mindful.**

Being mindful is to replace any negative thought or action resulting from your thought with something that is beneficial and good. Most likely your environment triggers your thoughts, therefore the first thing to do is change your environment so that your outcome can be changed.

3. Exercise.

Regular physical exercise increases the production of new brain cells and increases your levels of dopamine, which are released in your prefrontal cortex.[61]

4. Sleep.

The prefrontal cortex is sensitive to fatigue that is induced by prolonged hours of being awake.[62] So being sure to get the proper amount of sleep at set bedtimes will increase your frontal cortical activity.

5. Selection of food.

It has been shown that when one is obese, there is lower activation of the prefrontal cortex.[63] So consuming foods that lower the prevalence of obesity would consist of minimally processed whole foods such as:[64]

- Whole grains (whole wheat, steel-cut oats, brown rice, quinoa)

- Vegetables (a colorful variety-not potatoes)

- Whole fruits (not fruit juices)

- Nuts, seeds, beans, and other healthful sources of

protein (lentils, quinoa, and tempeh)

• Plant oils (olive and other vegetable oils)

• **What kind of selfishness do I naturally possess? Does that give me a true supportive connection?**

_____

_____

_____

• **How do I connect with my family and friends?**

_____

_____

_____

_____

• **Who can I connect with that will fill my social connection need and I will fill their need?**

_____

_____

ASK YOURSELF

As you are given this new day filled with 24 hours, how are you going to use it to benefit your social community around you? Not only should you practice unselfishness to those around you, but also it is vital to surround yourself with people who give something back to you.

CHAPTER 9

The Environment

"Know your environment. Protect your health."

– ENVIRONMENTAL WORKING GROUP

One of the most powerful things about regenerative self-care is that when you live it out in every grain of your life, you become an eco-action hero without even trying to be.

When you choose to protect your health, you are in return protecting the environment that you and others live in. Every product that you choose to consume or partake in gives you the power to make a variety of positive impacts from little choice like reducing waste to building healthier habits.

WHAT YOU DON'T KNOW CAN HURT YOU

Imagine with me that it is a lazy morning and you are whipping up your favorite breakfast on the stove in your favorite nonstick pan for easy cooking. For all you know, your pan does a pretty good job at cooking your meal and you have an easy clean up without much scrubbing to do.

You, of course, are a healthy individual with no major health problems and you eat your meal believing that your organic selection of food will keep you healthier longer. Yes, eating organic food lessens the amount of pesticides in your body and is for sure a sustainable diet option, but what would you do if you eat healthily and still happen to get sick either from prostate or ovarian cancer, kidney cancer, thyroid complications, or birth complications or infertility?[65]

What you don't know won't hurt you. Is that really true? If this was only as true as it states. For what you don't know *CAN* hurt you.

WHAT YOU DON'T KNOW *CAN* HURT YOU

Perfluorooctanoic acid (PFOA) and Perfluoroalkyl substances (PFAS) are long-chain manmade chemicals that are not easily broken down.[66]

They are termed as 'forever chemicals' for their long and damaging existence. The purpose of these chemicals is to repel grease in food packaging's such as pizza boxes, microwave popcorn bags, certain takeout boxes, and anything else that repels grease or water like waterproof clothing and nonstick cookware.

PFAS or PFOAs resist any type of breakdown both in the environment and in our bodies, therefore meaning that we ingest these harmful chemicals through the water we drink, the food we eat, and the clothes we wear.

Over some time, the longer that we ingest these chemicals, they begin to build up in our bodies with the result being seen in cancers, endocrine disruptions, birth complications, and even reduced effectiveness of vaccines.[67, 68, 69, 70]

There are a few documentaries that you can watch to become more aware about harmful chemicals such as, Overload: America's toxic love story, Dark Waters, and Erin Brokovich.

Select one area of your house or a couple of items that you use regularly that are loaded with toxic chemicals and look for healthier alternatives.

KNOWLEDGE ABOUT WHAT IS BEING DONE WILL HELP YOU

Why is this so harmful to you when you are cooking your breakfast meal?

Ironically enough, PFOAs and PFAS have been shown to decrease dopamine sensitivity in roundworms.[71] So, when you are eating your deliciously prepared breakfast in a pan coated with PFAS or PFOAs, your excitement and pleasure may be rebuffed and you may not enjoy it as much as you anticipated.

More importantly, though, on June 22, 2020, the final rule from Congress in the FY 2020 National Defense Authorization Act stated that importers and a products agency only requires notification of the use of PFOA and PFAS when it is solely present on the surface of their products.[72]

Therefore meaning that manufacturers don't have to disclose to consumers that they're using them as long as these 'forever chemicals' are not on the surface of any of their products. Yet, the contraindications from these chemicals are still present. Ninety-eight percent of participants in the Centers for Disease Control and Prevention's National Health and Nutrition Examination Survey detected PFAS in their bloodstream, breast milk, and umbilical cord blood.[73]

In 2015, there were hopes to make a change in how manufacturers disclose information to their consumers with the EPA proposing a Significant New Use Rule (SNUR).[74]

The intent for this SNUR was to prevent any of these chemicals to be present without the agency's knowledge and approval and also to prevent any new uses of the chemicals. What seemed like a short victory was overtaken by the Congress rule On June 22, 2020, where now once again most consumers are unaware of these 'forever chemicals' and to our detriment putting us at risk.

WAYS THAT YOUR CHOICES MAKE AN IMPACT

What can you do with the knowledge that you now have?

Here are simple ways that you can begin to incorporate into your daily routine and interactions that will limit your exposure to PFOAs and PFAS.

- Purchase products that are PFAS free or free of

fluorocarbons or fluorinated chemicals.

• Replace nonstick cookware with stainless steel, cast-iron, glass, or ceramic alternatives.

• Ask your water provider for data on PFAS testing in your area. If there has been no testing done in your area, ask your provider or state to start monitoring for these chemicals and install treatments to remove PFAS from your water.

• Avoid ordering or heating food that is contained in grease-resistant packaging.

• Make popcorn on the stovetop, in a stainless steel pot of course.

The power lies in you to know the information that you need to live a healthier life in a healthier environment.

Healthy living is about protecting your health as well as the health of your environment and planet. When you take care of your health nutritionally, you are aware of what chemicals are in your products, and you go back to nature, you are making an impact on a better environment. And when the environment is better, then the future generations will have a better chance at keeping your work going that you have started.

We live in a world where a tree is worth more dead than alive. If you do not use the power of your choice to change that fact, then your environment will be worse for the next generation. Your children will have a harder battle to fight.

Life just happens once. Be sure to do what is right in making your environment better for future generations.

CHAPTER 10

Money That Smells

"Money is like manure.
You have to spread it around or it smells."

– J. PAUL GETTY

I looked at that $2 bill in my hand with awe. It was so crisp, so new, and so much money all in one little piece of paper. My Grandma and Grandpa had given this $2 bill to me in my Christmas card, and to me, this was enough money to buy the whole toy store!

Growing up, we did not have that much extra money to spread around because of my Dad's hospital and medical bills, so any extra money that was given was a special treat.

Shortly after I had received that $2 bill, some people had come to town sharing what they were doing in a different country to help children learn to read and write. Something was tugging at my heart to give my new, crisp $2 bill to help those children. Even though I didn't have all the money in the world, I for sure had the privilege of learning how to read and write here in

America, plus I even had a backpack to hold my pencils and paper.

Instead of giving the only money that I had, I decided to keep it for myself and comforted my conviction by telling myself that $2 wouldn't do much to help those kids and I could instead buy the toy that I have been wanting. Those kids need much more than what my $2 bill would give.

That next week, as I went to look for my $2 bill, it was missing. I could not find it anywhere. I looked in my pockets, my closet, my drawers, the car, everywhere I looked for it, but it was nowhere to be found.

The conviction came again, but this time, it came as regret. I regretted not sharing my money for those kids. I was sad that because I chose not to listen to my first intuition to give to help others, now no one has the opportunity to appreciate the benefits that my crisp $2 could give.

NO AMOUNT IS TOO SMALL

No matter how much money that you have in your bank account or whether you just came back from a shopping spree, if your money is not used in a way that does not bring back a compound effect, it becomes smelly.

In 1937, at the time of his death, John D. Rockefeller was worth over $340 billion in today's money. Rockefeller did not always have this much money, though. He grew up in a humble country home in New York where he learned at age 14 the pivotal lesson of how money works.

He worked hard to save his first $50 and his mother encouraged him to lend his $50 to a local farmer with the arrangement that after one year he would be paid back with 7% interest.

A year later the farmer kept his deal and returned to Rockefeller his $50 plus $3.50 in interest.

It was then where Rockefeller realized that the $1.12 that he made in three days of digging potatoes in a field was less than one-third of the annual interest on his $50.

This lesson of learning how money can work for you is important. There are only so many hours in the day that you can put towards making a change in the world, so discovering how to use your money in a way that will do the work which you cannot do is important in your self-care routine.

In actuality, most people self-care with their money. Money that is used for self-care that does not bring back interest is smelly.

It used to be that you would feel better when you spent money on an item for yourself, like a purse, a pair of shoes, or other material goods. There is a sense of gratification and an immediate mood lifter when you buy something, yet after the fact, you would feel twice as guilty about spending money on material goods rather than spending your money on an experience.

There is now a movement towards spending money on experiences instead of items, which actually in turn can inspire positive changes in your community and the world when people come together and experience events.

Being mindful of where your money goes and thinking of how your money can work for you to bring back an interest can begin with knowing that all of your essential items are bought and taken care of. This is helpful to know so that when you do want to buy any material good that you already may have or do not need, then you can remind yourself to put your money into experiences instead.

IT'S OK TO BUY THAT DRESS

Most of us have the essentials for survival such as basic clothing, food, shelter, and water. So what do you do when your basics are covered, yet you still see a dress or an item that you want?

There are three things that I have taught my kids since they were able to walk, talk, and get dressed. When they choose their clothes in the morning they need to make sure that they are:

1. Weather appropriate.
2. Each clothing item matches the other.
3. Modest and covers all of your body parts decently.

Because they were taught this from the very beginning, I don't have to come after them constantly and tell them to put on a sweater, cover up their assets, or explain that orange plaid does not match with purple floral. It is a part of their lifestyle.

It's time to add a fourth one now that they are getting older and asking to buy more clothing.

4. Parents will buy essential clothing of their choice every season. If any other items are wanted, they may choose to save for that specific item if it follows the first three instructions.

There is nothing wrong with wanting something that is more than essential, nor is there anything wrong with spending something on yourself as a special treat.

What is wrong with that is when there are no boundaries. Boundaries for when it comes to what is budgeted for those extra fancies. For in actuality, most people self-care with their money. So focusing on how your money can bring a reward back to you is key in a regenerative lifestyle.

Money should be focused to buy necessary things with an occasional treat. Invest in bonding with your family and friends and focus on building memories that can last, rather than holding onto a $2 bill that could become smelly.

• **How much am I able to budget each month for my extra wants without spending over my income?**

_____

_____

_____

_____

ASK YOURSELF

• **What are things that I can do to encourage me to stay within my budget?**

_____

_____

_____

_____

WHAT TO DO WITH YOUR MONEY

Resources are limited in this world, and most people cannot have everything that they want, while others have more of what they want and need than others.

No matter if you have $1 or $1,000,000, here are four simple things that you can do with your money and resources that you have so that your money can work for you and bring back benefit.

1. **Save.**

   Money saved today is worth more than money saved tomorrow.

Life gives unexpected blows, so putting away a little bit of money every month will help you build an emergency fund to use for unexpected emergencies. This is not intended for last minute gifts, a needed spa treatment, or an enticing sale. This will alleviate the stress of not being able to pay for such emergencies.

2. **Invest.**

   The sooner you get going, the less you have to do.

Put resources, such as money, into an account or an organization for the purpose of growing the value and impact of the resources.

3. **Spend.**

   Create and stick to a budget by weighing your income vs. your expenses and your needs vs. your wants.

You have the power to spend when you want, where you want, and on what you want. The power also lies in you to make healthy choices with how you spend. To alleviate spending more than what you have, develop a written plan on how you can spend less than what you earn.

4. **Donate.**

Give time, talent, or monetary gifts with no expectation of something in return.

• **How much money do I make each month?**

_____

_____

WRITE IT

• **What are my monthly expenses? Do I have a budget that weighs my income vs. expenses and needs vs. wants that allows me to spend less than what I make?**

_____

_____

_____

_____

- **What are my financial goals that will give return over time?**

	Short-Term (1-3 Years)	Mid-Term (3-7 Years)	Long-Term (7+ Years)
Retirement income	☐	☐	☐
Buy new home	☐	☐	☐
Set up emergency fund	☐	☐	☐
Education Fund	☐	☐	☐
Support parents	☐	☐	☐
Start a business	☐	☐	☐

CHAPTER II

Self²

"Small, daily elevations compound into massive results over time."

– ROBIN S. SHARMA

The United States 16th President, Abraham Lincoln said, "That some achieve great success, is proof to all that others can achieve it as well."

This does not mean that how one person achieves success will be the same way that you achieve success. Success comes to you when you daily exceed who you were yesterday and strive every day to be better than before.

Little by little, the choices that you make in how you take care of yourself today, will transform you into who you have always wanted to be right now and tomorrow.

You will be transformed into a person who takes responsibility for their actions by being a:

- Convicted action promoter

- Aware of the weight of your choices

- Living with less regret

- Intrigued with the power that lies in you

- Inspired to make a change in people's lives

HOW DO YOU KNOW IF YOUR LIFESTYLE IS REGENERATIVE?

Everything is in harmony, you are fulfilled, and your action and choices give back for the better of yourself, your community, and the planet as a whole.

The last question that I had for myself in my regenerative lifestyle journey was what do I do with vacation? Something was missing and I knew that I hadn't fully reached that moment where my self-care habits had been squared exponentially.

I don't know how you vacation, but with my husband being Portuguese he loves to travel and explore, while I would be happy relaxing at the beach the entire time. It was through his passion to explore that it expanded my view on how vacations were done and helped me to answer the last question that I had.

Most of us go on vacation because we are burnt out at work, we need to recharge, or we meet with friends and family because we have missed personal connections.

The powerful thing with vacations is that if it is not done right, you can come back feeling the same or even worse than you were before you went. But, when vacations are done right, you cannot only see better results in your health, outlook, and improved performance, but you can also take advantage of squaring your results exponentially.

Here are four ways to exponentially square your vacation so that your actions can personally compound into massive results.

1. Giving you new ideas.

On our last vacation, my husband and I had an opportunity to go on a date without our little ones. What we weren't expecting was to spend an hour in a cute little bookstore, sitting on a comfy couch, perusing books of our choice. That special bonding time opened up my eyes to want to start a new project when I got home, while my husband got inspired to try a new recipe.

2. Broadens your horizons.

It's easy to forget that there is an entire world outside of your little town or even your home. When you travel to different places in the world, it opens your horizons to experience cultures that you would most likely not experience otherwise.

3. Connected to the community as a whole.

When you are not focused on your work, your home, and the small duties of life, you become more connected to those around you. Opportunities are more readily available to build lasting relationships when you are traveling and on vacation than if you were to be at home. You experience the life of others in their community and build a bond.

4. Vacation with a purpose.

Have a plan for what you will do when you go on vacation. Be sure to relax while still exploring the culture and surroundings. To make your vacation truly exponentially squared, plan a project that you will do to give back to the community that you are visiting.

When my family goes to Florida to vacation, we take time every morning or evening to walk the beach with gloves and a bag. By the end of our walk, our bag is full of trash that was missed by the beach patrol clean-up and would be a hazard to the ocean life. My daughter said, "I feel so good knowing that the birds and the animals that live in the ocean will not get hurt and die by this trash." She could not be more proud knowing that she left the beach a better place than when we found it.

• **How do I feel when I come back from vacation?**

_____

_____

_____

_____

ASK YOURSELF

• **What things/activities do I do on vacation that make me feel restored?**

_____

_____

_____

_____

• **What are some ways that I can vacation with a purpose?**

_____

_____

_____

_____

You now have the tools to produce compound results in your life by your daily choices and habits. How will you change your lifestyle habits to produce greater results?

CHAPTER 12.

Carpe Diem

"Opportunities come and go, but your spiritual vision is non-negotiable."

– DAVID BAYER

You can only change what you choose to and what you are convicted about. You can read this book and be inspired about all the powerful ways that you can be a healthier and happy person through regenerative self-care and you can wish to daily make a positive influence in this world and on those around you, yet not do anything about it.

Unless you are personally convicted, personally challenged, and personally affected by the changes, nothing will alter your current state of thinking. To transform who you were before reading this book to a convicted action-changing promoting lifestyle, you need to make a choice.

You now have the choice to make the change and live a life that you are intended to live that connects your mind with your body. Today is the day for you to choose. How will you choose to Carpe Diem?

In my life, I have attended more funerals than I have wished for, and most often there is read from the front, The Dash Poem by Linda Ellis.

I read of a man who stood to speak

At the funeral of a friend.

He referred to the dates on the tombstone

From the beginning...to the end.

He noted that first came the date of birth

And spoke the following date with tears,

But he said what mattered most of all

Was the dash between those years.

For that dash represents all the time

That they spent alive on earth.

And now only those who loved them

Know what that little line is worth.

For it matters not, how much we own,

The cars...the house...the cash.

What matters is how we live and love

Carpe Diem

And how we spend our dash.

So, think about this long and hard.

Are there things you'd like to change?

For you never know how much time is left

That can still be rearranged.

If we could just slow down enough

To consider what's true and real

And always try to understand

The way other people feel.

And be less quick to anger

And show appreciation more

And love the people in our lives

Like we've never loved before.

If we treat each other with respect

And more often wear a smile,

Remembering this special dash

Might only last a little while.

So, when your eulogy is being read

With your life's actions to rehash...

Would you be proud of the things they say

About how you spent YOUR dash?

There is sorrow at a funeral, yet also a realization that life is precious and too short. You are still alive right now. How will you live your life between the date you were born and the date when you pass away?

Your journey is as important as your legacy.

• **What do I want to accomplish during my life?**

_____

_____

_____

_____

ASK YOURSELF

• **Why is this helpful to others and me?**

_____

_____

_____

• **How can I make this dream a reality?**

_____

_____

_____

As David Bayer says, "Opportunities come and go, but your spiritual conviction is non-negotiable." What project have you been wanting to complete, what program have you been dreaming to sponsor, or what change in the world do you want to be a part of?

One Question To Help You Trust

What would you do if you knew that everything was going to be ok?

If you were to tell me right after I saw my Dad with a rope

around his neck that there was someone that I could trust, I would have rolled my eyes at you and told you to leave me alone.

And that is what happened.

I did not trust anyone or anything after this experience, not even my husband when we got married. It was only after I began to live this regenerative lifestyle of self-care and began to experience the benefit of my needs being met and my community being restored from my choices, that I began to trust fully in my husband and the community around me.

Whether you are a spiritual person or not, you have a spiritual conviction that is non-negotiable. What are you going to do with it? How are you going to trust that conviction to the better of yourself and the future?

I now know that no matter what goes wrong and what setbacks I experience, that the God that I trust will take care of things. To be honest with you, most times it is not taken care of the way that I expect it, but when all is said and done I trust that all things have worked together for the betterment of everyone as a whole. But I had to first experience complete renewal from my regenerative lifestyle and harness the power that lies in me to make the choices that help me thrive and leave this world a better place before I could trust that everything would be ok.

The reason why I have such trust in my God is that He does not force me to do anything. No one can make you do something, only you are responsible for the choices you make and the way that you act out your choices. He gives me the freedom to use the power that lies in me to become the woman of honor and usefulness, the power to choose to become the person that I am meant to be, and it is only myself who can feel the power that lies in me to choose to make this world a better place by my thoughts and actions.

It is when I use my power to choose in conjunction with trusting in my God, that I will be the most permanently successful. I can trust Him to be there when things do not go as planned.

IT IS YOUR TIME TO CHOOSE

You know that feeling you get when the red apple is on your desk in your third-grade classroom because you are the student of the week?

Ever feel like that is the most wonderful thing in the world? Until you begin to notice that it took such a long time for that apple to get to *your* desk, yet it seemed to reach your friend's desks more frequently... again and again?

Yup, my hand is raised on this one!

Although I may have never been the most brilliant kid in school or got to enjoy that beautifully prized red apple on my desk for more than that one quick fleeting week, I am thankful that time gives equal recognition.

If there is one thing that makes us all equal, that is time. Time has no respect of persons, yet it is through time spent that one can see a direct reflection of your quality of life.

Time doesn't favor anyone because of where you grew up. Time doesn't favor which religious group you are a part of. Time doesn't favor what nationality you are or what color of skin you are graced with. Nor does time have a favorite doughnut it likes to be bribed with. Time is here to give you a chance. Chance to allow you to make the change to be restored and nourish your soul with regenerative self-care that gives back.

Chance comes to everyone. A chance to choose.

Chances are given to you for you to choose whether or not you will respect your mother, stand up for what you believe in, and choose to follow that which is honest and pure. And once again, chance does not stop because of your socioeconomic status, your community ranking, or if you choose to sleep with one sock on. Chance is here for everyone to choose and grab hold of, no matter your baggage or previous life story.

As a third-grader, I can vividly remember thinking two things about that red apple and how it made me feel. The first thought was that I wanted to throw that apple in all its red glory out the window so that no one could enjoy it. Without a doubt it made me feel sad, hurt, disappointed, not good enough, shameful, and wanting to not try anymore to prevent the hurt of being let down when my attempt was not appreciated.

Yet, the second thought I remember telling myself was that even though I may not have had the joy of being commended as the student of the week more than once in the entire year, I was appreciated for something (to this day I don't remember for what). But that was enough to encourage me that red apples don't show your quality of life, it is what you choose to do with them and the choice you take with the chances that are given to you.

Today may be the last day you have the time and chance to choose your quality of life. How are you going to live? Who are you going to put your trust in?

Your car will eventually run out of gas or electricity with no reliable refill source. Your staple food item will be taken by others with the same need. Your home may be destroyed by a natural disaster or invaded by unwanted guests, but when you have a reliable source to trust, you will not be shaken by circumstance, sight, emotions, or feelings.

Take the time to choose today who you will follow and put your confidence in, and make the change to view yourself as the person you are called to be.

As our final days are completed, what we have left behind can either be deprived of vitality or restorative and beneficial for future generations.

What will you choose to do with the power that lies in you?

156

CHAPTER 13

5-Day Kick Start Guide

"Empathy and honesty may be more important to success and happiness than hours of algebra coaching or the positive reinforcement of smiley face stickers on your homework growing up and at your work level."

– ROBERT COLES, M.D. & DANIEL GOLEMAN, PH.D.

Day One: Being *TRUE* to yourself

T: Truthfulness.

Are you honest with yourself? Is your true identity being mingled and crowded with your peers? Is it being molded and shaped by what you are looking at in social media?

- Be honest about your long-term happiness. Do not settle for another person's identity. Instant gratification doesn't normally help you in developing who you are and being true to yourself in the long term.

What do you want for your long-term happiness?

_____

_____

_____

_____

R: Relationships.

In every relationship, you will feel pressure. Pressure from your parents to do one thing, pressure from your peers to do another, and pressure from your work to accomplish your task in a certain way. While at times you may feel pressure from these relationships, do not reject them altogether nor ONLY find your identity in them. Our relationships with our parents are our anchor, for it connects us with our culture. Our relationships with our siblings connect us to our history. Our support relationships like our friends and enemies connect us to our character. Ultimately, our relationships reveal our identity, heritage, and legacy.

> • When we assume a relationship with others that is not true to our identity, we can be placed in circumstances that are not pleasing nor trustworthy. We may think that it's not the cool thing to be identified with our parents, or your siblings are just a nuisance when you are trying to hang

out with your friends. But when we hide who we are and our true identity, most often we are sniffed out like a rotten egg.

Do you hide who you truly are for fear of revealing your true identity? What are relationships in your life that are not in alignment with your identity?

_____

_____

_____

_____

U: Understanding.

Our attitude plays a key role in being true to ourselves. We must understand the motives for why we do things. If what you are doing involves rebellion, peer acceptance, personal pleasure, greed, or self-importance, you must understand that these things only bring about a short-term high that will only be followed by a long-term low.

> • It is also beneficial to understand that some behaviors or habits can be habit-forming and harm your mental capacity and understand that even by doing these acts, our initial excitement will wear off. These pleasures only last for a season.

What behaviors or habits do I partake in that harm my mental capacity?

_____

_____

_____

_____

How can I change these habits? Who can I reach out to for help and accountability?

_____

_____

_____

_____

E: Example.

What if you knew that you were a part of something bigger? You have an effect that can ripple even after you have passed away. Morally responsible people care about the example that they set for others. Would you want your younger sibling or your child to live the same life that you are? You want people to follow your positive behavior, not your dubious behavior.

- Being true to yourself, or the concept of being authentic is actually beneficial for your mental health. It helps with aspects of your psychological well-being, vitality, self-esteem, and coping skills.

What legacy do I want to leave behind from my actions?

_____

_____

_____

_____

Day Two: Conformity

How much do you do things for yourself or for others? Do you wonder what others will think or do if you do what you truly have passion for? How do you act in your job setting, your personal schedule, food preferences, and relationships? Do you conform to other people's preferences or do you live out your convictions?

Evaluate yourself on a scale from 1-10 on how much you conform to other people, with 10 being the most conformity and 1 being naturally creative with your true identity.

You want to eat a quinoa salad because you are choosing to eat healthier, but your friend suggests eating pizza instead.

<u>Naturally Creative</u>   <u>Conformity</u>

1   2   3   4   5   6   7   8   9   10

☐   ☐   ☐   ☐   ☐   ☐   ☐   ☐   ☐   ☐

You know that you are fully capable to complete this assignment at work, but you let your more 'qualified' co-worker take it.

<u>Naturally Creative</u>   <u>Conformity</u>

1   2   3   4   5   6   7   8   9   10

☐   ☐   ☐   ☐   ☐   ☐   ☐   ☐   ☐   ☐

You want to change your habit of going to bed late so that you can feel more rested, but your roommate or partner asks you to watch just one movie with them.

<u>Naturally Creative</u>   <u>Conformity</u>

1   2   3   4   5   6   7   8   9   10

☐   ☐   ☐   ☐   ☐   ☐   ☐   ☐   ☐   ☐

While you should be flexible when conforming to preferences, you should be firm on principle. If you believe that your health would be at risk if you were to eat a fast-food pizza or you believe in the principle that you receive the best hours of sleep before midnight, then kindly suggest another option to set a date during the weekend where you can enjoy the movie in the day together and make your pizza at home so that the ingredients are healthier for you.

Day Three: Motivating Factors

Self-care is done to relieve stress and recharge you to continue your life and fulfill your daily demands and tasks. The motivator and the effectiveness of your self-care habits can vary according to your temperament. What may seem fun and exciting may not leave you feeling fun and excited.

I think that having a spa day is one of the most exciting things to do. Yet, even though it may be relaxing when I am experiencing it, I cannot wait to leave and take a quiet moment to stroll through the trees to fully recharge my body before going home. What may seem like a motivator for self-care may not give you the results that you are looking for.

Example:

Habit	Motivator	Effectiveness of Self-Care
Spa	Relaxing & Rejuvenating	Short term

Think of three self-care habits that you partake in on a common basis and measure them to see if those habits resonate with your temperament and are truly restorative.

Task   Motivator   Effectiveness of Self-Care

_____

_____

Task   Motivator   Effectiveness of Self-Care

_____

_____

Task   Motivator   Effectiveness of Self-Care

_____

_____

Day Four: Unique Interests & Talents

Deep down in you, you have a passion. You have a drive. You have this small voice telling you that you are valued, precious, and honored. No matter if it seems like they are covered with dust and rusty from being out of service, I want you to ask yourself what do you enjoy doing? What are interests that uniquely inspire you? What talents do you uniquely possess?

What are your unique interests?

_____

_____

What are your unique talents?

_____

_____

How can you incorporate your unique interests and talents into your self-care routine?

_____

_____

Day Five: The ABCDEFG's of Regenerative Self Care

If you fill in the rest of the alphabet, I would love to see what you come up with!

To fully understand how to be true to ourselves amid the clutter

165

of counterfeits in our society today and to thrive with regenerative self-care, come with me as we go through the first 7 alphabet letters to find out.

A: Attitude.

Having an attitude of what can I give, instead of what is best for me can give your more meaning and satisfaction than having everything that you have ever wanted monetarily.

What is something that I want right now?

_____

_____

Does that something benefit only me?

_____

_____

If this something benefits only me, how can I change my attitude from thinking this is good for me, to is this something that is truly necessary?

_____

_____

Can I live without this if I was only able to keep 3 essential items?

_____

_____

B: Behavior Control.

How do you respond in situations? Do you react in ways that you are proud of and are beneficial for yourself and others?

Create a buffer for yourself each day for the situations that are thrown at you that may alter your normal equilibrium. The best way to do this is to carve out a morning routine that fills your cup and gives you the ability to be more patient, understanding, loving, and kind.

What do I do for my morning routine that fills my cup, rejuvenates me, and gives me an extra cushion of patience for the day so that my behavior is one that I can easily control?

_____

_____

_____

_____

C: Concept.

Be honest about your self-concept.

> • How you see yourself is largely defined by what you believe the most important person in your life thinks of you. This is where you must implement truthfulness because what if the most important person in your life does not think highly of you, does not see the gifts and uniqueness that you have to offer, or puts you down? Attaching your self-worth to someone else's opinion may not be the honest concept of yourself. Be honest and true to yourself that no matter what you have been told, look beyond and see the value that you have to bring to this world that no one else has to offer except yourself.

How do you view yourself?

_____

_____

_____

_____

In what ways do you dream to increase your self-concept so that you can feel valuable and change the way that you see yourself from other's negative views of you?

Increase:

_____

Increase:

_____

Increase:

_____

Increase:

_____

Increase:

_____

Increase:

_____

D: Decision.

Decide if you want a happy life or a meaningful life. A happy life consists of taking from the resources available, while a meaningful life is giving back what you have taken in your unique way.

I decide to live a meaningful, regenerative life beginning today!
☐

Signed:

_____

Date:

_____

E: Example.

Would you be proud if others chose to do the same thing as you? Is the life that you are living morally responsible?

F: Future Destination.

What regenerative impacts do you desire to make in:

2 Years:

_____

5 Years:

_____

_____

10 Years:

_____

_____

20 Years:

_____

_____

G: Good.

Otherish Motivation, this is self-care beyond ourselves. Doing good for others gives us a responsibility to something greater than ourselves.

What program(s) do I want to be a part of?

_____

_____

What charity do I want to sponsor?

_____

_____

References

CHAPTER TWO: REWRITE YOUR STORY

1 • Shear M. K. (2012). Grief and mourning gone awry: pathway and course of complicate grief. *Dialogues in clinical neuroscience, 14*(2), 119–128.

CHAPTER THREE: THE REGENERATIVE PROCESS

2 • Ohlhorst, S. D., Russell, R., Bier, D., Klurfeld, D. M., Li, Z., Mein, J. R., Milner, J., Ross, A. C., Stover, P., & Konopka, E. (2013). Nutrition research to affect food and a healthy life span. *The Journal of nutrition, 143*(8), 1349–1354. https://doi.org/10.3945/jn.113.180638

3 • Harvard Health Publishing. (2018, May 1). Understanding the stress response: chronic activation of this survival mechanism impairs health. Retrieved from https://www.health.harvard.edu/staying-healthy/understanding-the-stress-response

4 • Yim, J. (2016). Therapeutic Benefits of Laughter in Mental Health: A Theoretical Review. *The Tohoku Journal of Experimental Medicine, 239*(3), 243-249. https://doi.org/10.1620/tjem.239.243

5 • Ágoston, C., Urbán, R., Király, O., Griffiths, M. D., Rogers, P. J., & Demetrovics, Z. (2018). Why Do You Drink Caffeine? The Development of the Motives for Caffeine Consumption Questionnaire (MCCQ) and Its Relationship with Gender, Age and the Types of Caffeinated Beverages. *International journal of mental health and addiction, 16*(4), 981–999. https://doi.org/10.1007/s11469-017-9822-3

6 • Budney, A. J., & Emond, J. A. (2014). Caffeine addiction? Caffeine for youth? Time to act! *Addiction, 109*(11), 1771–1772. https://doi.org/10.1111/add.12594

7 • CDC, NIOSH. (2020). Interim NIOSH Training for Emergency Responders: Reducing Risks Associated with Long Work Hours: Caffeine. Retrieved from https://www.cdc.gov/niosh/emres/longhourstraining/caffeine.html

8 • Temple J. L. (2009). Caffeine use in children: what we know, what we have left to learn, and why we should worry. *Neuroscience and biobehavioral reviews, 33*(6), 793–806. https://doi.org/10.1016/j.neubiorev.2009.01.001

CHAPTER FOUR: MIND BODY CONNECTION
9 • https://loni.usc.edu

10 • Breit, S., Kupferberg, A., Rogler, G., & Hasler, G. (2018). Vagus Nerve as Modulator of the Brain-Gut Axis in Psychiatric and Inflammatory Disorders. *Frontiers in psychiatry, 9*, 44. https://doi.org/10.3389/fpsyt.2018.00044

11 • Shu-Zhen, W., et al. (2010). Effect of Slow Abdominal Breathing Combined with Biofeedback on Blood Pressure and Heart Rate Variability in Prehypertension. *The Journal of Alternative and Complementary Medicine 16*(10). https://doi.org/10.1089/acm.2009.0577

12 • Lehrer, P. M., & Gevirtz, R. (2014). Heart rate variability biofeedback: how and why does it work?. *Frontiers in psychology, 5*, 756. https://doi.org/10.3389/fpsyg.2014.00756

13 • Gevirtz, R. (2013). The Promise of Heart Rate Variability Biofeedback: Evidence-Based Applications. *Biofeedback, 41*(3), pp. 110-120. https://doi.org/10.5298/1081-5937-41.3.01

14 • Shu-Zhen, W., et al. (2010). Effect of Slow Abdominal Breathing Combined with Biofeedback on Blood Pressure and Heart Rate Variability in Prehypertension. *The Journal of Alternative and Complementary Medicine 16*(10). https://doi.org/10.1089/acm.2009.0577

15 • Knoch, D., & Fehr, E. (2007). Resisting the power of temptations: the right prefrontal cortex and self-control. *Annals of the New York Academy of Sciences, 1104*, 123–134. https://doi.org/10.1196/annals.1390.004

16 • Shaffer, F., McCraty, R., & Zerr, C. L. (2014). A healthy heart is not a metronome: an integrative review of the heart's anatomy and heart rate variability. *Frontiers in psychology, 5*, 1040. https://doi.org/10.3389/fpsyg.2014.01040

17 • Blum, J., Rockstroh, C., & Göritz, A. S. (2019). Heart Rate Variability Biofeedback Based on Slow-Paced Breathing With Immersive Virtual Reality Nature Scenery. *Frontiers in psychology, 10*, 2172. https://doi.org/10.3389/fpsyg.2019.02172

18 • Porto, P. R., et al. (2009). Does Cognitive Behavioral Therapy Change the Brain? A Systematic Review of Neuroimaging in Anxiety Disorders. *Journal of Neuropsychiatry and Clinical Neurosciences, 21*(2), 114-125.

19 • Shou, H., Yang, Z., Satterthwaite, T. D., Cook, P. A., Bruce, S. E., Shinohara, R. T., Rosenberg, B., & Sheline, Y. I. (2017). Cognitive behavioral therapy increases amygdala connectivity with the cognitive control network in both MDD and PTSD. *NeuroImage. Clinical, 14*, 464–470. https://doi.org/10.1016/j.nicl.2017.01.030

20 • https://www.glycemic-index.org/high-fibre-diet.html

21 • NIH. (2012). Breaking Bad Habits: Why It's So Hard to Change. Retrieved from https://newsinhealth.nih.gov/2012/01/breaking-bad-habits

22 • Ratey, J. (2002). *User's Guide to the Brain* (New York, NY: Vintage Books) p. 17

23 • Popkin, B. M., D'Anci, K. E., & Rosenberg, I. H. (2010). Water, hydration, and health. *Nutrition reviews*, *68*(8), 439–458.https://doi.org/10.1111/j.1753-4887.2010.00304.x

24 • Helliwell, J., Layard, R., & Sachs, J. (2019). World Happiness Report 2019, New York: Sustainable Development Solutions Network.

25 • Tankersley, D., Stowe, C. & Huettel, S. (2007). Altruism is associated with an increased neural response to agency. *Nat Neurosci 10,* 150–151. https://doi.org/10.1038/nn1833

CHAPTER FIVE: LOCALLY GROWN
26 • https://fdc.nal.usda.gov

27 • Cryan, J., Dinan, T. Mind-altering microorganisms: the impact of the gut microbiota on brain and behaviour. *Nat Rev Neurosci* 13, 701–712 (2012). https://doi.org/10.1038/nrn3346

28 • https://www.ams.usda.gov/about-ams/programs-offices/national-organic-program

29 • https://royalsocietypublishing.org/doi/10.1098/rstb.2010.0172

30 • Nicolopoulou-Stamati et al. (2016). Chemical Pesticides and Human Health: The Urgent Need for a New Concept in Agriculture. *Frontiers in Public Health*. https://doi.org/10.3389/fpubh.2016.00148

31 • https://www.beyondpesticides.org/resources/state-pages/oh/school-policies

32 • https://www.researchgate.net/publication/49739590_Impact_of_Pesticides_Use _in_Agriculture_Their_Benefits_and_Hazards

33 • https://www.ewg.org/foodnews/#0

34 • https://www.ncbi.nlm.nih.gov/pmc/articles/PMC5551144/

CHAPTER SIX: PERSONAL CARE PRODUCTS

35 • Miller, K. (2021). *Endocrine Disorders.* WebMD. Retrieved from https://www.webmd.com/diabetes/endocrine-system-disorders

36 • http://www.lc-ms.nl/phthalates.htm

37 • Kamarina, C. (2019). *A-Z List of Toxic Chemicals Within The Glycol Ethers Category.* AZChemistry. Retrieved from https://azchemistry.com/list-of-toxic-chemicals-within-the-glycol-ethers-category

38 • https://www.publicgoods.com

CHAPTER SEVEN: THE NOT SO TYPICAL EXERCISE

39 • U.S. Department of Labor. (2021). *American Time Survey —May to December 2019 and 2020 Results.* Bureau of Labor Statistics. Retrieved from https://www.bls.gov/news.release/pdf/atus.pdf

40 • Vahratian, A., et al. (2021). *Symptoms of Anxiety or Depressive Disorder and Use of Mental Health Care Among Adults During the COVID-19 Pandemic – United States.* MMWR. 70(490-494). DOI: http://dx.doi.org/10.15585/mmwr.mm7013e2external icon

41 • Kahn, P., et al. (2009). *The Human Relation With Nature and Technological Nature.* Current Directions of Psychological Science. A Journal of the Association for Psychological Science. 18(1).

42 • Pearson, D. G., & Craig, T. (2014). The great outdoors? Exploring the mental health benefits of natural environments. *Frontiers in psychology, 5,* 1178. https://doi.org/10.3389/fpsyg.2014.01178

43 • Li Q. (2010). Effect of forest bathing trips on human immune function. *Environmental health and preventive medicine, 15*(1), 9–17. https://doi.org/10.1007/s12199-008-0068-3

44 • Keniger, L. E., Gaston, K. J., Irvine, K. N., & Fuller, R. A. (2013). What are the benefits of interacting with nature? *International journal of environmental research and public health, 10*(3), 913–935. https://doi.org/10.3390/ijerph10030913

45 • https://www.health.harvard.edu/mind-and-mood/is-an-underlying-condition-causing-your-fuzzy-thinking

46 • Thompson Coon, J., et al. (2011). Does participating in physical activity in outdoor natural environments have a greater effect on physical and mental wellbeing than physical activity indoors? A systematic review. *Environmental science & technology, 45*(5), 1761–1772. https://doi.org/10.1021/es102947t

47 • Randall, C. L., & McNeil, D. W. (2017). Motivational Interviewing as an Adjunct to Cognitive Behavior Therapy for Anxiety Disorders: A Critical Review of the Literature. *Cognitive and behavioral practice, 24*(3), 296–311. https://doi.org/10.1016/j.cbpra.2016.05.003

48 • Ribeiro Porto, P., et al. (2009). Does Cognitive Behavioral Therapy Change the Brain? A Systematic Review of Neuroimaging in Anxiety Disorders. *The Journal of Neuralpsychiatry and Clinical Neurosciences. 21*(2). 114-125. https://doi.org/10.1176/jnp.2009.21.2.114

49 • Hoffman, M., Hoffman, A. (2008). Exercisers Achieve Greater Acute Exercise-induced Mood Enhancement than Non-Exercisers. *Physical Medicine and Rehabilitation. 89*(2). 358-363. DOI:https://doi.org/10.1016/j.apmr.2007.09.026

50 • Prabakaran, S. (2015). Endocannabinoids Mediate Runner's High. *Science Signaling. 8*(401). 322. DOI: 10.1126/scisignal.aad7694

51 • Stathopoulou, G., et al. (2006). Exercise Interventions for Mental Health: A Quantitative and Qualitative Review. *Clinical Psychology Science and Practice. 13*(2). 179-193. https://doi.org/10.1111/j.1468-2850.2006.00021.x

52 • http://citeseerx.ist.psu.edu/viewdoc/download?doi=10.1.1.454.814&rep=rep1&type=pdf

53 • Sharma, A., Madaan, V., & Petty, F. D. (2006). Exercise for mental health. *Primary care companion to the Journal of clinical psychiatry, 8*(2), 106. https://doi.org/10.4088/pcc.v08n0208a

CHAPTER EIGHT: SOCIAL CONNECTION

54 • Crocker, J., Canevello, A., & Brown, A. A. (2017). Social Motivation: Costs and Benefits of Selfishness and Otherishness. *Annual review of psychology, 68,* 299–325. https://doi.org/10.1146/annurev-psych-010416-044145

55 • DeSteno, D., Bartlett, M. Y., Baumann, J., Williams, L. A., & Dickens, L. (2010). Gratitude as moral sentiment: Emotion-guided cooperation in economic exchange. *Emotion, 10*(2), 289–293. https://doi.org/10.1037/a0017883

56 • Boykin, A. W., Albury, A., Tyler, K. M., Hurley, E. A., Bailey, C. T., & Miller, O. A. (2005). Culture-based perceptions of academic achievement among low-income elementary students. Cultural Diversity and Ethnic Minority Psychology, 11, 339–50.

57 • Canevello, A., & Crocker, J. (2010). Creating good relationships: Responsiveness, relationship quality, and interpersonal goals. *Journal of Personality and Social Psychology, 99*(1), 78–106. https://doi.org/10.1037/a0018186

58 • Shu-Zhen, W., et al. (2010). Effect of Slow Abdominal Breathing Combined with Biofeedback on Blood Pressure and Heart Rate Variability in Prehypertension. *The Journal of Alternative and Complementary Medicine 16*(10).

59 • Knoch, D., & Fehr, E. (2007). Resisting the power of temptations: the right prefrontal cortex and self-control. *Annals of the New York Academy of Sciences, 1104,* 123–134.

60 • Christov-Moore, L., Sugiyama, T., Grigaityte, K., & Iacoboni, M. (2017). Increasing generosity by disrupting prefrontal cortex. *Social neuroscience, 12*(2), 174–181.

61 • Hauber W. (2010). Dopamine release in the prefrontal cortex and striatum: temporal and behavioural aspects. *Pharmacopsychiatry, 43 Suppl 1,* S32–S41.

62 • Muzur, A., Pace-Schott, E. F., & Hobson, J. A. (2002). The prefrontal cortex in sleep. *Trends in cognitive sciences, 6*(11), 475–481. https://doi.org/10.1016/s1364-6613(02)01992-7

63 • Gluck, M. E., Viswanath, P., & Stinson, E. J. (2017). Obesity, Appetite, and the Prefrontal Cortex. *Current obesity reports*, 6(4), 380–388. https://doi.org/10.1007/s13679-017-0289-0

64 • Harvard, School of Public Health. (2020). Obesity Prevention Source. Retrieved from https://www.hsph.harvard.edu/obesity-prevention-source/diet-lifestyle-to-prevent-obesity/

CHAPTER NINE: THE ENVIRONMENT

65 • Strassner, C., et al. (2015). How the Organic Food System Supports Sustainable Diets and Translates These into Practice. *Frontiers in nutrition*, 2, 19. https://doi.org/10.3389/fnut.2015.00019

66 • https://health.ri.gov/water/about/pfas/

67 • Chang, E., et al. (2014). A critical review of perfluorooctanoate and perfluorooctanesulfonate exposure and cancer risk in humans. Critical Reviews in Toxicology, 44(1) DOI: 10.3109/10408444.2014.905767

68 • Ballesteros, V., Costa, O., Iñiguez, C., Fletcher, T., Ballester, F., & Lopez-Espinosa, M. J. (2017). Exposure to perfluoroalkyl substances and thyroid function in pregnant women and children: A systematic review of epidemiologic studies. *Environment international*, 99, 15–28. https://doi.org/10.1016/j.envint.2016.10.015

69 • Savitz, D. A., Stein, C. R., Bartell, S. M., Elston, B., Gong, J., Shin, H. M., & Wellenius, G. A. (2012). Perfluorooctanoic acid exposure and pregnancy outcome in a highly exposed community. *Epidemiology (Cambridge, Mass.)*, 23(3), 386–392. https://doi.org/10.1097/EDE.0b013e31824cb93b

70 • Grandjean, P., Budtz-Jørgensen, E. (2013). Immunotoxicity of perfluorinated alkylates: calculation of benchmark doses based on serum concentrations in children. *Environ Health* 12, (35). https://doi.org/10.1186/1476-069X-12-35

71 • Sammi, SR., et al. (2019). Perfluorooctane Sulfonate (PFOS) Produces Dopaminergic Neuropathology in *Caenorhabditis elegans*, *Toxicological Sciences*. *172*(2). 417–434. https://doi.org/10.1093/toxsci/kfz191

References

72 • https://www.congress.gov/116/bills/s1790/BILLS-116s1790enr.pdf

73 • Calafat, A. M., Wong, L. Y., Kuklenyik, Z., Reidy, J. A., & Needham, L. L. (2007). Polyfluoroalkyl chemicals in the U.S. population: data from the National Health and Nutrition Examination Survey (NHANES) 2003-2004 and comparisons with NHANES 1999-2000. *Environmental health perspectives*, *115*(11), 1596–1602. https://doi.org/10.1289/ehp.10598

74 • https://www.federalregister.gov/documents/2015/01/21/2015-00636/long-chain-perfluoroalkyl-carboxylate-and-perfluoroalkyl-sulfonate-chemical-substances-significant

Acknowledgements

To my husband, who is supportive in all of my crazy ideas and passions, whether they are successful or not. Your love amazes me!

My precious jewels, my children, who have inspired me in more ways than you will ever know.

My Mom, who's support and love has been like a rock, and to Francis who has treated me like his own.

I am thankful to my sisters for every fight, every tease, and every exchange of love.

My mentors who saw something in me and pushed me to be more.

To my friends who have been an intricate fabric in my regenerative self-care journey.

Special Thanks To

Rebecca Cafiero

As one who likes to give credit where credit is due, I could not pass up this opportunity to shine the light on a very special and amazing individual. Rebecca has not only written the foreword to this book, but she has taught me that writing a book is not just about putting words on a piece of paper, but rather it's about leaving your footprint in the world through your own unique and special way. She has definitely left an impactful imprint in my life and if you want to experience a portion of her sincerity, genuine character, knowledge, and gentle guidance, join The Pitch Club Goal Getters Facebook Group where she and her team work hard to provide valuable resources for female business owners and entrepreneurs who want to work for themselves but not by themselves. Your life and the legacy you leave behind will never be the same.